To my wife Barbara,
our daughters Amy and Camille,
and our granddaughter Alma.

TABLE OF CONTENTS

Preface.. 3
Introduction 7
Acknowledgements 25
About the Author... 27
1. Growing up in Asia... 29
2. People Who Helped Shape my Character While Growing Up....... 59
3. Uncle Siu & Aunt Pauline – My College Education 87
4. Adulthood in America..................................... 95
5. My First Big Business Intrigue – Protein from Petroleum.......... 111
6. Herbalife – My First Experience with Multi-Level Marketing 119
7. MLM Cookies Corporation – The Company of Diet Cookies 131
8. David vs. Goliath: NCI SBIR Phase II Database Contract, What if…? 139
9. Adulteration Continues to be a Major Problem.................... 145
10. Michigan Alumni Distinguished Lifetime Achievement Award 151
11. Dietary Supplement Label Database (DSLD) – Not for Herbal Supplements 155
12. What is Wrong with Drugs and Herbal Supplements........... 161
13. Proper Modernization of Chinese Medicines.................... 181
14. What Should We Do with our Invaluable Herbal Treasure?...... 195
15. Glossary & Abbreviations 205

PREFACE

Two main reasons have prompted me to decide to tell my story:

First. It's for my daughters (Amy and Camille) and granddaughter (Alma) to know something about my family background and what I have done so far in my life, as there are no close family members around for them to consult. For years, my daughters didn't even know what my profession was. Their friends' fathers might be chemists, pediatricians, accountants, nurses, or engineers. But their father is a pharmacognosist...what? No one is sure what that is.

During my professional career, I have dealt with botany, chemistry, drugs, herbs, hallucinogens, hallucinogenic mushrooms, Chinese medicines, Chinese tonics, single-cell protein from petroleum, fermentation, and opium alkaloids, among other scientific matters. All of which are within (or claimed to be within) the realm of pharmacognosy. One year I was a chemist, another year a microbiologist, and yet another year a Chinese herbalist; my career was like a chameleon. How do you explain that to your daughters? Especially when even most pharmacognosists themselves don't quite exactly know what their own field is, and the word pharmacognosy is often not even listed in dictionaries. Furthermore, once I found it listed in one of the popular dictionaries, it was defined as a part of pharmacology.

I often wonder how that came about, and how many pharmacologists under forty years old in the world have even heard of the word pharmacognosy, let alone have studied it. However, some of them, eighty years or older, may have heard of materia medica, the field from which both pharmacognosy and pharmacology are derived. But as far as I know, pharmacognosy was never a part of pharmacology. On the contrary, some pharmacognosists may actually study the pharmacology of natural materials. For example, my studying the culture of *Psilocybe* fungi and the chemistry of the hallucinogens they produce might easily lead to the study of how some of these hallucinogens may work to reduce stress or to help treat mental illnesses in humans.

So, I don't blame my family for not being able to tell others what my profession is, because it would take a chapter to describe what it is or is not. In fact, I have already written about this puzzle sixteen years earlier in my Newsletter, *Leung's (Chinese) Herb News* [LCHN] in Issue #32 (May/June 2001) under the title, "Pharmacognosy Revisited." [This LCHN is being simultaneously republished in book form along with this Memoir. See **LCHN**[1]]

Second. I have grown up with traditional Chinese medicine and have personally experienced the effects and benefits of Chinese herbs and formulas. My family and I still use numerous traditional formulas from China (available in America for many decades) for common ailments such as flus, colds, coughs, hay fever, pimples, canker sores, and other aches and pains, as well as to maintain good health. You'd understand why as you read more of my story and in **LCHN**. I have also conducted scientific research on herbs (including Chinese herbs) and observed their trending towards chemical drugs for forty plus years. And only during the last twenty did I finally start to realize that scientists, including myself, for over 100 years, have all been using the same wrong technologies, those developed specifically for chemical drugs, whenever we want to investigate traditional herbs.

Scientifically, there is nothing wrong with singling out a particular chemical in any herb and trying to turn this chemical into another drug, one which carries with it none of that herb's documented traditional indications, safety, benefits, or other attributes. However, in doing so, we fail to utilize the herb's often copious recorded traditional data, data that could benefit us in the many areas where modern drugs fail us. This herbal (botanical) information can be found nowhere else. And because of this fixation on pure chemical drugs, we have increasingly neglected the true value of traditional Chinese herbs. The end result is

---

1 LCHN = Leung's (Chinese) Herb News, simultaneous republished with this Memoir

that, for at least a few decades now, we have missed the opportunity to achieve better health for fellow world citizens. We have failed to take advantage of the rich human experiences extensively documented in the traditional Chinese medical literature, which are still in use today. Instead, it is painful to watch the modern drug influence on scientists (especially those of Chinese descent), which is now so pervasive that most of them are following the chemical-drug path. They look down on TCHM[2] as backward and without merit, and treat traditional Chinese herbs inappropriately, as only chemicals or chemical sources.

Instead of letting traditional Chinese herbs continue to serve primarily as a cheap source of modern chemical drugs, I want to preserve them. During my career of at least fifty years, I have never seen Chinese herbs properly evaluated. They have been studied using the scientific technologies specifically developed only for chemical drugs, not complex herbal medicines or food. Consequently, results obtained have been equivocal, generating much controversy throughout the past decades, prompting many scientists to denigrate Chinese herbs and herbal practice as non-scientific and full of mumbo jumbo. But the fact is, many such studies had not even used the right herbal materials!

Hopefully, my continuing work and message can reach the influential people in China and other Asian countries with significant Chinese populations, where traditional Chinese herbal medicine is not yet 'fatally' compromised by modern drugs. This select group most likely doesn't even know that one of the major treasures of our Chinese heritage, TCHM, has been exploited for decades by the pharmaceutical industry and its followers (now including dietary supplement companies). It has been exploited to such a critical point that we are about to lose its well-documented relevance. If we don't stop this chemical trend, in another generation, Chinese herbs as they have been known and documented over millennia, may no longer exist. This is because some of them, like *zhiheshouwu* (cured fo-ti, a famous Chinese antiaging tonic), are now produced, not based on traditional practice, but on some spe-

---

2 TCHM = traditional Chinese herbal medicine, traditional Chinese herbs, Chinese herbs, Chinese medicines

cific chemical that is now required to be present in <u>both</u> the toxic raw fo-ti and the nontoxic cured fo-ti. This chemical was absent (or present in only trace amounts) in the traditionally cured fo-ti less than fifteen years ago, before this chemical requirement took effect as listed in the Chinese Pharmacopoeia of 2005. If this chemical trend continues, the whole documented treasure of Chinese herbs and formulas will be relegated to historical museums. Years from now once we wake up to this fact, its contents will no longer be relevant or useful for obtaining truly modernized herbal products. By then, it will be too late.

Being a perpetual optimist, I still have hopes that once these influential people are cognizant of the rapid disappearance of true TCHM, something will happen to reset the pharmaceutical industry's influence. Hopefully, it will lead to the readjustment of the thinking of those scientists and technical experts to reassess their views and positions. This will be for the health benefits of billions of world citizens, rather than for the continued self-enrichment of those who seek profit over healthful, nontoxic, natural treatments.

I have already started the basic step to modernize TCHM the correct way, which will retain its historical tradition. This is not based on some assumed active chemical, but on each herb's total attributes as traditionally used and documented. With this as a start, I hope a new industry based on truly modernized TCHM can serve as a new source for non-toxic and safer alternatives to modern drugs. True herbal supplements based on Chinese herbs and formulas, not on some specific chemicals, can serve as a start. I hope some members of the newer generations, those with honesty, bright brains, and compassion, will pick up this idea and build a new industry to serve the public.

INTRODUCTION

The following e-letter serves to introduce the main professional part of my story. It was sent over four years ago, as is, to about 250 colleagues and friends who held important positions in industry, government and academia. Most of them had earlier subscribed (or access) to my Newsletter, *Leung's (Chinese) Herb News* (ISSN# 1523-5017), published between 1996 and 2004, in which I frankly and honestly discussed practically all major issues relating to herbal medicines, including supplements. And many of them have been quietly supporting my continuing efforts in trying to tell the truth about herbs and the issues causing their ongoing problems. Many of these issues are still relevant and unresolved today, though they continue to be discussed by experts (real or self-proclaimed) as if they just came up yesterday.

OPEN LETTER TO COLLEAGUES AND FRIENDS
REGARDING HERBAL SUPPLEMENTS

October 29, 2013

Dear Colleagues/Friends,

Politics aside, the scientific state of healthcare in our country is not good, especially in the preventive area. Twenty years ago, it was American consumers' demand for alternatives to chemical drugs that had led to the establishment of the Office of Alternative Medicine (which came and went), Office of Dietary Supplements (ODS), and National Center for Complementary and Alternative Medicine (NCCAM). However, after having spent billions of our tax dollars over this period, we are <u>not</u> providing consumers with the true herbal alternatives (e.g., supplements) they seek. Being alternative only in material source, these chemical-based supplements have no connection to traditional usage other than the names of their source botanicals. They also have no prior safe-use history, because their safety assessment in humans, as with conventional drugs, only begins from the time they are put into clinical use following successful clinical trials.

I have devoted over 50 years of my professional career to the identity and quality of herbal products. Hence, it has been frustrating <u>to see not only inappropriate science being used on traditional herbs but also marketing hype and expediency often trumping scientific truth.</u> Nowadays, whoever speaks the loudest or being the most visible is often considered the authority delivering the truth, irrespective of his/her real expertise or insight in the subject. It's now the 21st century, yet preventive medicine continues to be equated simply to the early detection of diseases, so that they can be treated symptomatically with drugs. Nutrition and herbal supplements, two of the key areas that can actually strengthen the body and improve health to prevent diseases in the first place, are generally ignored or slighted by the medical and scientific establishments at large. Marketers and scientists involved in these fields are enabled to maximize profits and to seek the most expedient path, i.e., treating and promoting supplements as if they were drugs, ignoring their potential health-improving benefits as commonly believed and for which they have been traditionally used over centuries. Unless this trend is reversed soon, we would not have another chance to provide consumers with true alternatives to conventional drugs. Instead, <u>only arbitrarily selected chemicals that easily meet conventional drug criteria</u> (e.g., identity, quality, action) will be produced. Yet no one seems to be concerned enough to address this issue, even among my esteemed colleagues. Their focus and efforts are still being mostly concentrated in trying to develop and produce 'active' chemicals (sold as nutraceuticals, phytochemicals & supplements) which offer nothing alternative other than their non-synthetic source.

We need to have the courage to make some fundamental changes to the way science is being inappropriately applied to traditional herbal medi-

cine so as to provide consumers worldwide with the true alternatives to toxic chemical drugs which they deserve.

*Respectfully,
Albert Y. Leung, Ph.D.*

The Dietary Supplement, Health and Education Act (DSHEA) was passed in October, 1994, because American consumers wanted to have continued easy access to herbal medicines that they had already been taking for decades. Tired and wary of the toxic side effects of modern chemical drugs, they had chosen herbs (especially Chinese herbs) as an alternative, and didn't want them to be taken away under potential new regulations. These regulations would treat herbs as chemical drugs or food additives requiring prior approval before being put on the market, as threatened by the Food and Drug Administration, which would severely restrict their access. The DSHEA has essentially placed some herbal medicines in the supplements category, now known as herbal supplements, and legally treated as food. The belief is that since these herbs have been used for centuries (some, millennia), they come with the human experience of safety and benefits as traditionally known and handed down from generation to generation. That is a valid concept.

However, since the passage of the DSHEA over 20 years ago, herbal supplements have been treated right from the start as drugs and not as food. I think the reason is that there were no scientific technologies for adequately dealing with herbs other than those specifically developed and used for drugs. So, the wrong science has been used on these multi-component herbs since day one, generating many meaningless or ambiguous results, hence much controversy. Yet all the time scientists have been calling results from research studies on herbs 'non-scientific' and 'cannot be duplicated.' They are literally correct because, unbeknownst to them, they have been using the wrong science that has given them ambiguous, irrelevant, or irreproducible results. How can this kind of drug science produce relevant scientific results with herbs? It is no different than asking an electrician to fix a complicated plumbing problem in your home and expecting the problem to be solved. Most likely, it will not be. At best, the solution is not dependable, because you have used the wrong kind of professional. Then you declare the plumbing problem uniquely unfixable because the faucet continues to drip. For many decades, this has been the problem with the handling of herbs using the wrong science.

That is not all. Besides the wrong handling of herbal supplements as drugs, there is more with modern drug therapy that renders it no more scientific than the practice of herbal medicine, especially TCHM. This reminds us that the practice of traditional medicine has been mostly an art, relying on the skill and experience of the doctor. Only in recent decades have we started calling drug therapy (a predominant part of the current practice of medicine) scientific, while other treatment modalities like TCHM, non-scientific, and not 'evidence-based,' despite the latter having been with us since human history began and co-evolving with us over time. Even an isolated chemical from herbs has a history with us, and is at least not brand new to this earth, like a new synthetic drug whose toxicity is totally unknown.

The reason a new synthetic drug has to go through all the initial testing *in vitro*, *in vivo*, and so forth, is to be sure it is not so toxic as to kill living animals, before being subjected to human testing in clinical trials. And only then does its human experience actually start. Compared to the practice of TCHM whose human experience started thousands of years ago (probably causing misery and death during the first few hundred years or more), the modern drug therapy's human experience only starts now, comparable to the budding phase already experienced long ago by the practice of TCHM. There is no science that can bypass this human-experience phase. In our modern era, we are doing nothing new or 'scientific' in our modern drug therapy other than reinventing the wheel.

Finally, and most importantly, there is one last thing which we seem to have neglected to consider. It is our <u>body</u> during the human phase of drug therapy. It is not just one visible variable. We are all in fact unique individuals with extremely complex bodies, each of which is composed of countless chemicals, cells, tissues, and a myriad of other living matters, all working independently and in concert. None of our bodies is exactly like the others. Disturbance in one area most likely reverberates throughout our entire body. Imagine a chemical drug that enters our body to supposedly neutralize some target or block some enzyme assumed to be responsible for our problem, but it immediately meets a sort of chaos (though highly organized and living as far as our body itself is concerned). And is it supposed to go directly to the targeted chemical or cell without bumping into any one of the millions of other potential targets and not causing havoc? Good luck! I am a scientist, but I am confused about how this supposedly 'scientific' process works. If you make a brand-new chemical, no matter how scientifically, and introduce it into our infinitely complex and living body without some means (scientific or artistic) to direct it straight to your assumed (chosen) target, but, instead, let it fend for itself trying to make its way through millions of potential targets to the one(s) you have picked, how scientific is your drug therapy process with so many uncontrollable parameters? I suspect this is the reason why <u>all</u> drugs have side effects, whether they are a single chemical, synthetic or naturally derived, because no one can predict how much havoc they will cause before they reach their target(s). And since we can't change our body, we have to work with it. It is obvious to me that our TCHM system, having had prior contact and experience with our body, would work better with it than any brand-new synthetic drug (whose toxicity is totally unknown) which has at most only decades of contact experience with our body.

With the above basic facts on synthetic drugs and natural herbal therapies, along with our body's eventual involvement, let's put the relevant facts in proper perspective to see how science may play a role in medicine, modern or otherwise.

Basic science is normally one constant and one variable at a time, so that you can observe the changes among variables. It's not one constant and two or more variables all at once; or worse, two (or more) constants and two or more variables all at once. Then it would be impossible for us to observe the changes. Nevertheless, all these happen in our modern 'scientific' and 'evidence-based' drug therapy <u>as well as</u> in 'non-scientific' herbal therapies. These are not science but simply random events. It's difficult, if not impossible, to measure the results.

Let's take the following three scenarios that are taking place right now around the world:

1. A drug (a constant) enters the human body that at first simply appears to be one visible entity, but is in fact a highly organized living complex of countless chemicals, cells, tissues, and others (i.e., many variables all at once, not one at a time). In such chaos, do scientists know how to direct this drug to bypass millions of chemicals or cells to go straight to its targeted enzyme or receptor (or whatever they assume to be the culprit) to neutralize it to resolve our problem without disturbing other parts of the body? I highly doubt it. Just look at the dozens of side-effects of <u>any</u> drug listed in fine print in its package insert! Where can these side effects come from? I have tried to figure out, but options are few. They all eventually ended up in the uncontrollable nature of our body that is chaos to the drug, causing an unpredictable scenario, as I've already described.

2. Consider the above scenario but replace the drug with a true herbal supplement. Unlike the drug, this herbal supplement does not have only one single chemical, it has many, countless, in fact. Now, instead of one constant, it has multiple, and all together. When it enters the body, you have a situation that appears to be worse than the first. It is not the result of scientific planning or strategy; it is by chance. Consequently, to accomplish the process of modern drug therapy, we need the artistry and skill as well as the experience of the physician more than anything else. That's why we used to call traditional herbal medicine art, and correctly so. We never called it scientific because it's more like gambling than science. Only during recent decades did we start calling the major part of modern medicine (i.e., drug therapy) scientific. However, it is far from scientific, as long as the drugs have to go into the complex, totally uncontrollable yet highly organized 'mess' that is our body!

   Nevertheless, with a TCHM material that is similar to, and sometimes actually is, a food (fruit, root, leaf, seed, and other forms), we have already had thousands of years of experience with it. It may not be scientific or 'evidence-based' medicine or whatever you think sounds fancy to awe consumers and others, but we have prior experience with it innumerable times since antiquity. We also have practical knowledge and documented evidence that it works, so we do not need to treat it like synthetic chemical drugs that require toxicity testing from the ground floor. However, we have so far failed to utilize this human experience to our benefit, but have instead adopted modern synthetic drugs with totally unknown safety records. So we try to make sure they are suitable and not too toxic before putting them to work in humans. On a scale of human history with herb use spanning thousands of years, it was only about 3,500 years ago (give or take 500 yrs.) that documented history of Chinese herbal medicine began. The first documented record on Chinese drugs, *Wu Shu Er Bing Fang* (*Prescriptions for Fifty-Two Diseases*) around 3,000 years ago, already described over 100 toxic drugs (herbs, minerals & animal) that obviously our ancestors continued to use knowing that they were toxic. Then, about 1,000 years later, the *Shennong Ben Cao Jing* (*Shennong Herbal*) appeared, the first book exclusively devoted to drugs, describing 365 drugs, grouped into three categories: superior (nontoxic), medium (potentially toxic, depending on use), and inferior (toxic). It had taken probably thousands of years of human experimentation before our ancestors knew what kills, what hurts, and what is safe by the time they started writing their experiences down. And it has been an ongoing process since.

The fact is, the information is there. We know what to take and what to avoid. And just like foods, we need not use 'evidence-based science' to test whether or not they are safe for us to ingest, because our antecedents have done most of those tests for us over a period of millennia. Some toxic ones were reclassified as safe, and some safe ones have required added cautions. There is no need for us to start all over, as with some totally new chemical such as a synthetic that has never been tested. With this new synthetic drug, it may take a few hundred years before we consider it toxic and file it away, or if safe, it may become something like a TCHM such as astragalus root, documented for at least 2,000 years now as a safe tonic (i.e., used both as food and medicine). The fact is, no science can simplify or shorten this human-testing process as long as we have our current extremely complex but well-functioning body, containing billions of chemicals and cells. Hence, neither of the two scenarios is scientific. Both are art. The second scenario with TCHM has already been tried and true, yet no one has taken advantage of it. Think what the world can gain using natural therapeutics, instead of using toxic drugs that beget new diseases. These diseases in turn require new toxic drugs to counter, in a perpetual vicious cycle that only benefits the pharmaceutical industry and interdependent parties, but continues to harm the public and generate more patients. Remember, no one can change our body to a single entity with measurable characteristics to make our human drug therapy process <u>scientific</u>.

3. With the human body unchanged, containing umpteen variables (chemicals, cells, and tissues), we now replace the drug or true herb with <u>some herbal material</u>, let's call it 'something'. This 'something' could be some isolated chemical(s) or an extract prepared not according to traditional methods but based on the assumption that the herb contains some chemical(s) that <u>may be</u> (but highly unlikely) responsible for all its properties and effects known or documented for centuries or millennia. These 'something' supplements constitute a major part of what are sold and marketed today as herbal, or simply, dietary supplements. This is the group of herbal supplements which contains some products marketed as herbal, but with nothing from the advertised herb except a couple of chemicals <u>supposedly</u> from it. The constituents in these products are so varied that two products on the market from two different companies, with the exact same herbal ingredients on their labels, can be different as night and day.

Unlike the first two scenarios, the 'something' of the therapeutic part in this third scenario can be anything - a single chemical, two or more pure chemicals, extracts with high concentrations of chemicals but nothing else herbal, or one or two standardized chemicals with no relevant herbal elements in them whatsoever. The reason I call this category of dietary supplements the 'something' supplements is because, other than with some pure nutritional chemicals (such as vitamins, minerals, & amino acids), the herbal ingredients in these 'something' supplements can contain anything. While during the past few decades there have been considerable efforts and publications aimed at the identification and standardization of herbs and botanicals, little or no efforts have been devoted to the finished (processed) products. It is great we have the right herbs well-identified and standardized. However, unless there is absolutely no profit incentive in the step from raw botanicals to the finished products, how are we sure that the product manufacturer will actually put the right herbs there or use them in making their extracts? All these details on the raw materials (herbs) look good in theory and on paper, but they don't affect the quality of finished herbal products. My question is: Would any of these well-identified and standardized herbs be in the finished products? My answer is maybe. It can be also answered by the following question. Why am I still making my expert colleagues uncomfortable by talking about the identity and poor quality of herbal products, after having been in the herbal industry for decades and observing the inner workings of its product development and production, as well as the unethical or clueless practices of some players? I have also written about this in my Newsletter (**LCHN**), and in my books and other publications so many times over the past forty years. It makes me begin to sound like a broken record.

In any case, when you look at any herbal product label, the herbs listed don't mean anything. Although there are identity and purity standards for chemicals, all of which are analyzable, there is none for herbs. The reason is that there are still not even official guidelines for identifying and measuring herbal ingredients (except maybe the raw botanicals before processing, as I have just mentioned), let alone standards for them. My suggested comprehensive guidelines, first published in 1999 and reprinted in 2001 of my Newsletter, seemed to have fallen on deaf ears. Consequently, despite the efforts and the leadership of American Herbal Products Association (AHPA), and organizations like the USP/NF and AHP, companies still market <u>many</u> products with uncertain herbal ingredients. [see **LCHN-19 & LCHN-35; Chapter 9: Adulteration Continues...; Chapter 11: DSLD...**]

When you have such a 'something' supplement, you can neither depend on art nor science to assess it. It is basically a totally new <u>unknown entity</u>. None of the accumulated experience and wisdom of traditional herbs can help, because it is not one of them. Nor is it a known and well-defined chemical entity like a drug, so the science part of drug therapy can't help either. Consequently, when the unknown 'herbal' entity enters the body, anything can happen.

However, since decades ago when the herbal industry started, its profit-obsessed players, especially some newcomers, learned how to make sure their products were safe, by not adding too much of the herbs in their products. It appears to this day, this *modus operandi* is still followed. This means that the unknown herbal entity in scenario number 3 would be at least not likely to be too toxic when a wrong herb happens to be used.

For years, I have advocated cleaning up these products because consumers spend much of their hard-earned money to buy these products that afford them no health benefits, and only strain their finances.

Several years before I lost my business to imitation (adulterated) products, we developed a comprehensive fingerprinting method as part of our Phyto-True system. This technology was used for analyzing my own products and commercial products to assure the herbal products were genuine, and not just some standardized chemicals or inert fillers. That was twelve years ago.

The Phyto-True system was developed as a by-product of a Small Business Innovation Research (SBIR) grant from the National Center for Complementary and Alternative Medicine (NCCAM) in 2001, now renamed National Center for Complementary and Integrative Health (NCCIH). The grant was for investigating feverfew's antimigraine ingredients, and was awarded to my company with me as the Principal Investigator and Dennis V.C. Awang, Ph.D., as my Co-principal Investigator. Please note the name change again; this time from NCCAM to NCCIH. It seems my colleagues in charge are still trying to grapple with justifying the variable results of using the wrong technology in treating herbal medicines as chemicals while they are actually regulated as foods.

A few years back, our Food and Drug Administration started to use similar fingerprinting technology to make sure commercial herbal products are what they claim to be. [see **Chapter 9: Adulteration Continues...**]

This is the part of commercial herbal supplements that can be easily cleaned up with our fingerprinting technology if consumers are really interested in saving money and getting real herbal products that come with hundreds or thousands of years of human experience.

I am 80 years old. Having observed the increasingly irreversible trending of herbs to chemical drugs for more than thirty years and seeing no signs that anything is being done about it (in industry, government, or academia) I have decided to make one last try. I am now turning to the general public to inform them about how they have been increasingly supplied herbal supplements that are not what consumers had originally wanted. Many are not really herbal, but instead chemical, in a base of inert carriers, as the New York State Attorney General's Office had discovered by serendipity* (see **GLOSSARY**) and made public in early 2015. As consumers of herbal products (aka herbal medicines, herbal supplements, etc.), we want real herbal products that are tradition-based and have a true connection to their long-use history. We don't want chemicals in an inert matrix of fillers or carriers, marketed to us as 'herbal' supplements.

Over decades, I have repeatedly appealed to my colleagues who are involved in the research, production, and marketing of these products to consumers, urging them to be truthful to consumers in their work. The above e-letter was my last attempt almost five years ago. But again, there were no signs of anything coming from them, except that our FDA finally started a few years ago to require more comprehensive analyses of herbal ingredients in herbal products. Now, instead of only measuring a couple of chemical markers in herbal products or herbal supplements, the rest of the product's content is also analyzed, to avoid easy adulteration with unwanted fillers.

The FDA's starting to fingerprint the rest of the herbal components besides the marker compound(s) using a technology like our Phyto-True is a good start. But it will not reverse the products with standardized chemicals which at the present still meet legal requirements, as this 'legal' part is up to individual interpretation. There is no requirement to analyze all herbal components of herbal supplements besides their contents of some standardized marker chemicals.

We had been using Phyto-True fingerprinting for my own products years before our patent application. My papers on this technology were published between 2008 and 2010. With Phyto-True, we started the basic step in what I believe is the correct scientific approach to exploring the true nature and values of systematic traditional medicines like Chinese medicine. It is based on both tradition and science, not just blindly applying drug technology to a holistic system by zeroing in on some specific chemicals. These chemicals often have no relevance to the traditional nature of the herb/medicine, generating wrong, or at best, inconsistent results. But I need the public to understand the whole issue, and to demand that their herbal supplements be true and genuine, and not what they are increasingly becoming – chemicals disguised and sold as herbal supplements, or sold legally as dietary supplements.

Don't let the experts bamboozle you into believing that this herbal supplement business is so complicated that you, without sophisticated scientific training like theirs, are not supposed to be able to understand it. Yes, you may not understand the complexity of how a chemical structure is determined or how we can take a gene from a microbe and put it into an animal to change some part of that animal's character. But as a person with common sense, you can understand that trying to fit a square peg snugly into a round hole won't work. Likewise, it won't work trying to apply chemical technology meant only for pure chemicals to complex herbs with multiple chemicals, many of which are not even identified. For scientists with doubts, this is analogous to trying to understand what each line on our fingerprint means before accepting it as a unique part of our whole fingerprint that gives us part of our identity.

So, before taking any herbal supplements, be aware of what is present in them. Find out if it is standardized to (or only based on) any marker chemical that is often totally irrelevant to the properties and benefits for which the herb is traditionally known to have. It's fine if the herbal product contains traditionally made extracts standardized to some analyzable chemical(s), but it should also have other components normally present in the herb extracts as shown by relevant fingerprints.

At present, our original true herbal products/supplements have been trending towards chemicals (drugs) to such a point that the only way we can acquire real herbal products is to either make them ourselves, or seek out smaller companies that are more likely to still be making them. But then as a consumer, how do you know which ones to trust? After all, some small companies are not run or owned by knowledgeable herbalists, but instead by opportunistic businessmen. So, knowing exactly whom to trust, and which products are genuine, is unfortunately not currently feasible for most of us.

However, we can try to shame the marketers and purveyors of fake herbal supplements into starting to manufacture and sell genuine and good-quality products. We can do this by actually analyzing their products and showing the world how dismally lacking some of these products are. Any analyzable chemicals without herbal elements marketed as 'herbal' supplements would be easily revealed to consumers, and thus could be avoided. I also believe most of these businesspeople have been misled like many of us, and will come around when they are clearly shown the true nature of their products. This can put the opportunists out of business and prompt the ignorant but well-meaning producers/marketers to seek help in shaping up their product lines.

Having been intimately involved in the herbal industry most of my professional career, I have seen it all. I know exactly where to look for fake products. Several of my colleagues/friends and I have been considering setting up an organization (probably non-profit) to analyze these 'herbal' supplements using our Phyto-True technology to show consumers what these products actually are. Our organization will have the technical and business expertise, as well as the integrity, along with a competent participating lab, to accomplish this. We need you, and many of you, to be with us as friends and/or financial partners. We don't want to take away the chemicals/drugs from those of you who actually want them and may need them, especially before safer and better alternatives are available. But you should know the difference between chemical drugs and herbal medicines and formulas that have been safely and effectively used for centuries, especially Chinese herbs that often have extensive written records. The latter are the true alternatives to toxic chemical drugs the DSHEA of 1994 had originally intended to afford us, not the same toxic chemical drugs. They can be a major part of our health care, and can truly help us maintain optimal health, as well as restore it when we become ill.

I am a scientist and entrepreneur by nature and training. I have published books including my *Encyclopedia of Common Natural Ingredients Used in Food, Drugs, and Cosmetics* (John Wiley & Sons), that was first published in 1980; 2nd Edition in 1996, and its latest 3rd Edition, renamed *"Leung's Encyclopedia of Common Natural Ingredients Used in..."* was published in 2010. For eight years between 1996 and 2004, I also published 42 issues of my **LCHN** (now simultaneously republished with my memoir in book form) which has had a positive impact on the identity and quality of herbal products and on the quality of herb research. In addition, I have published dozens of technical papers on herbs, including a relatively new one on the proper approach to the investigation of traditional Chinese herbal medicine – the Phyto-True system. For better or worse, I can't keep my mouth shut when I see injustice being done, especially in areas that I know would hurt others' health and wellbeing, as well as their pocketbooks.

About nine years ago, after I lost my business to cheap imitation products (see **Chapter 9: Adulteration Continues...** and **LCHN**) to which my major client had switched, I had them analyzed side-by-side with my original products. I found the imitations to contain barely any herbal ingredients. Yet my name and likeness are still being used today on the Internet to promote their products as if nothing has changed. When the FDA's fingerprinting requirement is eventually in full force, hopefully with the interest and support of American consumers, this kind of 'herbal' supplement will not be produced, maybe in another five to ten years.

Finally, the reason I have consistently and purposely picked traditional Chinese herbal medicine (TCHM) and not Ayurvedic or other ancient medical systems to represent traditional therapeutics, is that TCHM is arguably the most scientifically advanced, as well as the least compromised so far by the pharmaceutical industry. They are also the most aggressively promoted natural products worldwide by Chinese companies. Unfortunately, these products are not the traditional kind, but the misguidedly 'modernized' kind that concentrates on arbitrary chemicals that are touted to represent TCHM. For example, ginsenosides are used to represent any ginseng and tetrahydroxystilbene glucoside (a compound closely related to resveratrol - a highly touted antioxidant present in wine) is used to represent both the toxic raw fo-ti (*heshouwu*) (1.0%) and the antiaging tonic, cured fo-ti (*zhiheshouwu*) (0.7%). Many of us know that resveratrol is a strong antioxidant. The current fad is antioxidants just as the fad in the 1950's and 1960's was alkaloids. It's fine, as fads come and go. However, the current fad, if sustained, would adversely affect the supply of genuine TCHM, using at least cured fo-ti as an example. If not checked, when we finally come around to realize Big Pharma's technologies are enabling the marketing of chemicals from TCHM, causing changes in the basic nature of our TCHM raw materials, we would not have the right herbs to start modernizing TCHM, even if we wanted to.

Throughout my Memoir and **LCHN**, I try to emphasize the fact that traditional herbal medicines are different from modern drugs (synthetics): the former have been present in our ecosystem since life began on our earth, while the latter are something totally new, whose toxicity is largely unknown. In drug therapy or herbal therapy, we have no scientific control of the environment inside our extremely complex body once either a chemical or a mixture of chemicals (i.e., herb) enters it. Only skill and experience of the healers count, along with time! Decades of experience with drugs are nothing compared to centuries and millennia with natural therapies, especially TCHM. I want my colleagues, if you happen to read this, to give the above some serious thought while putting yourself on a non-pharmaceutical mode. You can greatly contribute to helping our fellow consumers achieve better natural health by not following the same path of toxic drugs and drug-related diseases, in a perpetual vicious cycle that mainly benefits the pharmaceutical industry and its dependent businesses.

In my Memoir, you can read about my background and upbringing, as well as my failures and successes, in chapters that include information on the following:

- Early years – childhood to adulthood
- Flunked out of elementary school, then again out of high school
- Handicaps, including why my father called me 'Idiot Boy'
- Key people in my life besides family who have helped make me who I am, including my mentor in college, Padre Marcelino Andreu
- Taste of first big business intrigue – microbial protein from petroleum
- Jack of all trades
- Got fired from the only two regular jobs that I have ever had
- The DSLD is useless for telling product identity and quality of herbal supplements
- What does 'Modernization' of Chinese herbal medicine mean?
- Wrong research approach perpetuated by Big Pharma

- David vs. Goliath - beating the best-known expert in the world and his team in his own game - NCI database Phase II proposal, what if...?
- Probably being the first alumnus who initially declined an alumni lifetime achievement award from the University of Michigan
- Business failures

ACKNOWLEDGEMENTS

I consider my **Memoir** and Newsletter (**LCHN**) the most important records of my lifetime achievements, despite their narrative sometimes being politically incorrect and frank; it emanates from the bottom of my heart. They cannot be simultaneously published today without the help of many people who have crossed my path during seventy-seven of the eighty years of my healthy and vigorous life. These two books would have been published at least two years earlier if not for a rear-ender by a reckless female driver at a red stop light. That has caused me at least two years of my productive professional and social life, as well as yet undetermined numbers of my remaining years to have to continue physical and psychological therapy to deal with its aftermath.

These books would not have been published without the support of countless individuals who have been a part of my life. Among them, the first person I wish to thank is my wife, Barbara Haas Leung. She understands my handicaps and for almost fifty years of our married life, she has taken care of much of our family affairs, thus allowing me to concentrate on my work and writing. Unlike me, she is an efficient multitasker who, if born a generation or two later, would have been one of those smart power-women who run multinational corporations.

I wish to thank my sisters Mai Leung Thayer and Lilly Leung Ho for some of the information of our family background; and to Dr. Ambrose So for information about my father which I didn't have earlier.

I can't thank my grandma, mother, and amah (Ah Shun) enough for their patience in taking care of me while I was a child growing up in Asia when I was living in my own world and then later tolerated my many nonintentional actions or mischiefs that might have caused them much grief during my preteen and early teen years.

Also, without my core support group during my college years at the National Taiwan University, I would not have become a pharmacognosist and disruptor of the misapplied scientific technologies used in herbal supplements today; my sincere gratitude to all of them, especially Howard Hong-Kee Hou, Kwok Hong-Nin, Georgiana Hou (nee Liu Siao-Ju), and Nancy Lee (nee Ma Ying-Chee).

There are many colleagues and friends whom I would like to thank for their collaboration and support during my career of fifty plus years in natural products and related fields. However, because of my reputation as an open critic of some powerful segments of the drug and herbal industries, it may not be beneficial for some of these colleagues and friends to be openly known for supporting my views. Hence, I am not listing your names; but you know I have always sincerely appreciated your support. However, I want to thank my competent personal assistants at our former home office in Glen Rock, New Jersey, MaryAnn Schneider and Ellen Buckey. They worked for me for years until I lost my business. They took care of everything that I couldn't handle with ease, allowing me to concentrate on the R&D and production aspects of my company, Phyto-Technologies, Inc. My sincere thanks go to Darin Smith, Sue Benedickt, and my lab crew that included Heather Conway, Shannon Ehlers, David Hansen, Craig Hopp, Peter Zhang, and Pat Mettler, among others, for their dedicated work for many years. For those associates whose names do not appear here but who have been part of my life, you can find my words of appreciation in the text whenever appropriate.

Last but not least, I want to specially thank a few individuals who have been with me on this publication project from the beginning, for their encouragements and support, especially their continuing comments and advice. They include Diane Lawton, DuWayne Peterson, Mark Wdowik, William Dewey, and my daughters, Amy and Camille.

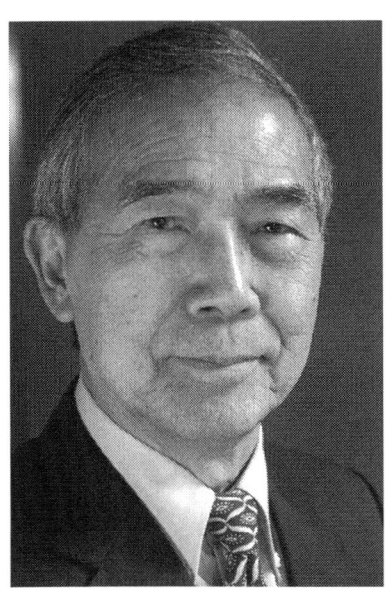

ABOUT THE AUTHOR

Dr. Leung is the original author of the *Encyclopedia of Common Natural Ingredients Used in Food, Drugs, and Cosmetics* (Wiley-Interscience) published in 1980, the Second Edition in 1996, and the Third Edition in 2010, renamed *Leung's Encyclopedia of Common Natural Ingredients Used in Food, Drugs, and Cosmetics*, by the same publisher. He is also the creator of PHYTOMED, a prototype computer database on Chinese herbal medicine developed under contract with the National Cancer Institute. Between 2000 and 2005, through an SBIR grant from NCCAM awarded to his company (Phyto-Technologies, Inc.), he and his team developed the Phyto-True system for properly handling complex herbal medicines with him as the Principal Investigator. Its analytical aspect is now beginning to be widely used for herbal supplements, a first step towards conducting meaningful scientific research on true traditional herbs and formulas.

CHAPTER 1

Growing up in Asia

MY FAMILY BACKGROUND

My Chinese name is Leung Yuk-Sing, Leung being my surname, meaning pillar, and Yuk-Sing my given name that means Sun-Rise. In Mandarin or *Putonghua* (common dialect), it is pronounced quite differently as *Liang Xu-Sheng* even though the written characters are the same. I was baptized a Catholic in college in Taiwan by Padre Marcelino Andreu, a Castilian Jesuit from Spain. He helped me pick the name, Albert (meaning bright), to go with my Chinese given name "Sunrise." Since "Albert" is also the name of my heroes – Albert Einstein in science and Albert Schweitzer – a humanitarian, missionary, and organist from the Alsace, we decided it was a perfect choice. Now, my full name is Albert Yuk-Sing Leung. In Hong Kong, it would be customarily written as Albert Leung Yuk-Sing. I am an American citizen since the early 1970's.

I was born and raised in Hong Kong. Both of my parents came from Guangdong, the coastal province in Southern China which abuts Hong Kong. My father, Leung Bing-Fun, was born in the city of Wai Chow (*Huizhou*), northeast of Hong Kong, now about 3 hours' drive from Hong Kong. My mother's maiden name was Ng Sui-Lan; she was born in the village of Mun Lau (*Wenlou*) in *Xinhui* county, northwest of Macau about a 2-hour drive from there. Neither of my ancestral towns is more than 75 miles or so from Hong Kong. Yet when I took my whole family along with a couple of close friends and business associates from the Dominican Republic (Jaime Dajer and his wife Marielle Duchatellier) to visit both my parents' birthplaces in 1989, it took us, in a hired van, with a driver, all day (7 or 8 hours) to get from Macau to *Wenlou*. The reason is that in those days there were no superhighways. Since *Wenlou* village is located in the *Zhuhai* (Pearl River) delta, we had to cross numerous strips of water by ferry to get there. The ferry had no schedule. It just waited until it was full before beginning the crossing to our side. Then, it would wait till it was filled up again before we would cross to the other side. However, the trip from Hong Kong to my father's city Wai Chow (*Huizhou*) was much faster, as we did not have to cross any water by ferry.

Both my parents' families were quite well-off. My paternal grandfather made part of his fortune in Malaya (now Malaysia) during the 1800's, I was told. His Third Wife was a Chinese woman from there, who was my grandmother. However, that part of my family history is so complicated that I have different versions of it and I have no idea which is totally true. The version that my father told me two or three years before he passed (in a 3-page letter of tiny scribbled Chinese) described our family history from his grandfather's generation to his father's and then his own. Both his grandfather and father had been cultured scholars and officials of the Qing Court. They each had at least three wives and many children. My grandfather was Number 8 among my great grandfather's children. My father was No. 9 amongst Grandfather's children. According to my father, Grandfather was an official in *Huizhou*. He also had a construction-materials business run by his fifth son, one of my father's older brothers from Grandfather's First Wife, who was a good-hearted woman to whom my father would turn whenever he needed advice or got into trouble. She was basically the family matriarch. This Fifth Brother of my father's was at least 25 years older than him. Around the turn of the century, in the early 1900's, the revolution was brewing and the society unstable; chaos abounded. At that time my father was only a little child, maybe a couple of years old, and my grandfather's favorite. He took the whole family including the First Wife, my grandmother (his Third Wife), my father, his older brother (child Number 7), and a younger sister (child Number 10) to Malaya to stay with my grandmother's clan. They all came back to *Huizhou* a few years later when my father was five years old and things in our home town had quieted down. He grew up going to a traditional Confucius school. At home, Grandfather taught him calligraphy and painting, along with Confucius philosophy and ethics befitting our family tradition. Unfortunately, when my father was thirteen, Grandfather suddenly died.

His Fifth Son (my Fifth Uncle) who probably had never learned much ethics from Grandfather, grabbed most of the inheritance. My father's Seventh Brother came home from Malaya and advised my father to live with Grandfather's First Wife. He took my grandmother (his mother) back to Malaya. This Seventh Uncle was the one who paid for my father's high school and college education after Grandfather died. He sent my father to Shanghai so that he would be far away from what we now would call a dysfunctional family. Seventh Uncle was the one Grandfather had sent to England to be educated there and later became an engineer. He had a son before he left for England. He later worked for Shell in Malaya in some high position and married an English woman. They had two sons. After this uncle died (was murdered, I was told), his wife went back to England with their sons. We may still have some cousins with the name of Leung living somewhere in England.

My grandfather was not only a scholar, teaching my father painting and calligraphy, he was also scientifically inclined, instilling in my father the love and respect for science. Consequently, besides being an amazing painter, at one time when he was in his sixties, my father experimented and succeeded in accelerating the production of sea salt using a simple solar process that drastically shortened the drying time. However, despite his friends in high places in Thailand, Malaysia, and Taiwan, he couldn't break the salt monopoly in those countries.

My father was also quite athletic. When he was in his teens going to high school and then to one of the most prestigious universities, Fudan University, in Shanghai, he was on the university's basketball and tennis teams. Other than that, I have no idea what else he did at college; and he never graduated because of his Seventh Brother's sudden death, leaving him with no more financial support for his education. However, he made a lot of loyal friends because of his extreme generosity and loyalty, to such an extent that he sometimes neglected his own family. In Hong Kong, especially among the Cantonese, we would say he had "yi hay" (*yi qi* in Mandarin). Once friends with you, the people with *yi qi* would stick with you through thick and thin and ask for nothing in return. I never met my paternal grandfather or grandmother. But I have met some of my father's rich and powerful friends. However, because of my personality, I never knew or cared much about schmoozing with any of them. After my father died, at the age of 90 or 91 (depending on how he counted), I don't remember any of them, except Dr. Stanley Ho Hung Sun and his protégé Dr. Ambrose So Shu-Fai whom I have met a number of times. My father always respected cultured and educated people and spoke highly of both, especially Dr. So who is years younger than I, but is well known as an erudite Chinese scholar fluent in both Putonghua and Cantonese as well as expert in calligraphy. He also speaks fluent English and Portuguese and is a top businessman in Hong Kong and Macau, running SJM Holdings, one of the businesses of Sociede de Jogos de Macau (SJM) started by Dr. Ho. When my father was alive, I noticed that Ambrose was always respectful of him, and took care of his needs whenever the occasion arose. I think it's probably because my father and Dr. Ho were friends, with my father being some years older than Dr. Ho, and Ambrose being a classic Chinese gentleman raised to respect elders.

After World War II and the communists having taken over China, my father lost his business around late 1940's and early 1950's and was never able to regain his footing, even with help from his loyal friends in high places in various projects in different Asian countries. The salt project was the only one I remember. Also, I was told by a couple of his friends that he was involved in the underground during the Second World War while I was living in my mother's village (*Wenlou*), active in breaking through Japanese lines to interact with Kuomingtang (Nationalist) agents. I have no way to verify that because my father's friends of comparable age are no longer around.

For the last few decades of his life, he hung out at the Hong Kong Chinese Recreation Club, a very exclusive club that cost a small fortune to join. He told me that Dr. Ho got him a free membership for life (probably Dr. Ho paid for it). No matter, after visiting Ambrose in Hong Kong recently, to confirm a few facts about the environment in which I grew up, I now realize my father could have gotten a lifetime membership years before he lost his business, and years before Dr. Ho even became a member.

Ambrose told me that the main reason Dr. Ho and my father were such good friends is probably because my father helped elect him President of the Chinese Recreation Club (CRC) decades earlier when Dr. Ho was running against another billionaire by rallying members behind him. Dr. Ho won and became the Club President. In any case, my father was often active in committee work as far as I could tell; and for years Dr. Ho and he were frequent tennis doubles partners at the Club. I know this because my father used to send me photos taken of him and Dr. Ho standing next to each other at the net holding their tennis rackets, or photos of them at some official function, decked up in tuxedos. He also at times sent me announcements of the Club which had his name or picture in them. This happened when he was up to his early eighties. The Club was like his second home, and he used to go there almost every day, even during the last few years of his life. Without the Club and his friends he would have been gone many years earlier. I thank both Dr. Ho and Ambrose for having played an important role for being his friends in enabling my father to live a more peaceful life in his final decades. I remember meeting Dr. Ho only three times, once at the Club, and once with my wife at his office in Hong Kong. The third time was at my product launch during the 1980's in Hong Kong. As to Ambrose, he provided the political and social connections for me, in the early 2000's, in my attempts to modernize traditional Chinese medicine the right way, not taking some chemical from traditional herbs and calling that modernized Chinese medicine. I was the only key scientist trying to direct modernization away from the easy commercialization of Chinese herbal medicines based on some assumed active chemicals supposedly holding the traditionally known and documented attributes of these herbs which are no different from conventional chemical drugs. [see **Chapter 13: Proper Modernization...**]

The family history on my mother's side is much simpler. As far as I know, there were no Imperial Court connections. My great grandfather was a village doctor serving his village and, I assume, nearby towns as well. There has been no mention among family members of his having more than one wife. And there was no family compound like that of my father's family next to the West Lake in *Huizhou,* which was destroyed during the Second World War by bombs, along with the Leung family businesses. I never even saw my father's house, or remains of it, except for part of the family business location during our family-history trip to China in 1989. A nephew, one of the grandsons of my Fifth Uncle (the selfish one) showed us where it was or could have been. A main street now ran through it and our business properties would have been spread across the road to both sides.

In contrast, my mother's family home was just a good-sized house with an open courtyard in the middle, and two wings, front and rear. Next to the rear wing was an open courtyard with a well and bathroom (not the modern kind) on one side, the backdoor leading to the outside was in the middle and the other side was the kitchen. The whole family (seven or eight of us) occupied rooms in the front wing, maybe also a room in the rear wing. In the middle facing the courtyard was a big room with two floors, I think. It was a mystery. We never dared to go in there. Perhaps that was where some of our ancestors' belongings were kept. I never asked. Once, I swear I saw an animal with scales there. I can't be sure, because I was five or six then, and there were so many ghost stories thrown at us by amahs and maids in my childhood that I was not sure it was real. I never knew what a pangolin or armadillo looks like until after I was in the United States and saw pictures of these animals in an animal book. The scaly animal I saw was a pangolin that I never saw anywhere else afterwards until I recognized it in the book. It must be real. But why in my Grandma's house?

Anyway, my maternal grandfather made his fortune in Havana, Cuba. He was a smart young man, smart enough to be the sau choi (*xiu cai*) of his region – meaning having scored high in some Imperial examinations that could lead to positions at the imperial court if he continued taking and scoring high in those exams to the national level. I am seriously lacking in the knowledge of Chinese traditions; and even this *xiu cai* thing is only story from my own family 'gossip.' I have no idea how Grandfather actually did in relation to the route leading to be an official in the Imperial Court system.

Obviously, my paternal grandfather and great grandfather must have scored high in the imperial exams to have attained the medium-level official status of 4th grade and 5th grade that would be comparable to our modern status of mayor and governor. That was according to my younger sister, Lilly. Now when I think of it, maybe that's why my older sister, Mai, somehow has come to own an ink stone belonging to the famous Chinese poet, So Tung Po (*Su Dongpo*) who lived in *Huizhou* around West Lake for a few years during his exile from the Emperor's Court for his outspoken views. Around the 10th and 11th century, *Huizhou* was considered southern-barbarian territory. But after Poet *Su* had written many poems extolling the beauty around *Huizhou* and its West Lake, it probably became a not-so-wild territory anymore by the time my family was living there 600 to 700 years later. We are Hakka or "guest families." My father spoke Hakka; so did Aunt Pauline [see **Chapter 3: Uncle Siu & Aunt Pauline...**], but none of us children speak it. Legend has it that we are Hans of central China but were driven down south into 'southern-barbarian territory' by the Mongols (Kublai Khan) when they established the Yuan Dynasty in the 13th century. We are now spread out in the southern provinces of China, and south-east Asian countries. According to a family legend, we are all supposed to have a deformed toenail on each of our little toes, which appears split and not smooth throughout. And I do.

In any case, back to my mother's family. During that time, Grandfather Ng (*Wu*) was in his late teens, and most of the young men who went to America to seek their fortune were from his region, especially Toy San (*Tai Shan*). But why did Grandfather go to Havana? I can only conjecture. My guess is he got on the wrong boat and somehow ended up in Havana. Or maybe being one of the extra adventurous young men, he decided to go to a less-traveled path and went to Cuba. There, he became a successful entrepreneur before returning to Hong Kong to await his grandchild's (my older sister Mai's) arrival in 1936, and later for good in the early 1950's not long before the Cuban revolution. He left his businesses, now including a Chinese herb shop, a supermarket (at first I thought it was a restaurant), and a laundry in the care of younger cousins. But as the Cuban revolution was brewing, his cousins started leaving for the U.S. and elsewhere and there was less and less money coming home. Before Grandfather came home for good, he also left his Cuban wife behind. I never met her but saw a photo of her with Grandfather; she was a lovely Cuban lady of Spanish descent.

When my wife and I took a tour of Cuba on an American Museum of Natural History 'study' trip in 2003, I took half-a-day off by myself to visit Havana's Chinatown to see what I could find out about my grandfather's business and Cuban life. I inquired about grandfather's restaurant (the "Golden Dragon or El Dragon de Oro" stuck in my mind) and his Chinese drugstore or herb shop, Wai Yuk Tong (*Hui Yu Tang*). But I was told that no such restaurant existed there. Then I met an old Chinese man on the street who happened to be the printer and editor of the only Chinese newspaper in Havana. He never met my grandfather, but he knew the name of my grandfather's herb shop, *Hui Yu Tang*, that happened to be right next door to his print shop. It was boarded up as condemned property and was quite deep, not a small place. He also confirmed that my grandfather didn't own any restaurant called the Golden Dragon. Later my younger sister, Lilly, who, along with Mai, are our family historians of sorts, told me it was not a restaurant but a supermarket. Anyhow, according to the newspaper editor and printer, there were only a hundred or so unassimilated Chinese left in Havana. The rest had married Spanish or Creole Cubans and moved elsewhere with their children. And my grandfather might have moved and lived elsewhere in Cuba with his Cuban family. In any case, at least as the only boy and 'heir' to my grandfather's fortune (if there were still one), I was able to personally get a glimpse of Grandfather's herb shop, a part of our family's lost fortune.

How Grandfather Ng ended up in Havana, Cuba, is still a mystery, especially when one of his peers and friends from the same village made his fortune in the U.S., I was told. Both had supported the village school and the village had built two classrooms in their honor, one for each. We saw them when we visited the school on that family trip in 1989 and then again when my sister Lilly and I visited our amah (Lilly and Mai's) only a few years ago at the same village. Their carved names were prominently displayed above the entrance to their respective classrooms. I distinctly remember a couple of things about my grandfather's friend and peer from his village (Granduncle Ng). He was a fat guy with a big belly. For a short time he and his family lived in Hong Kong after they returned from America. For whatever reason, he wanted to show us how to eat the American way. I was probably nine or ten years old. He took me and my sisters to a Western restaurant. It was my first time ever using a fork and knife. I don't remember the food or how we managed to eat it. But I do remember the occasion.

Since my mother was the only child of Grandma and Grandfather, she was dearly loved and must have gotten anything she wanted. She was smart with numbers and was sent to boarding school in Canton (now *Guangzhou*) run by Baptists, and from there to Shanghai to attend college – the same one my father attended (Fudan University), according to Mai. At that time, there were few women who attended college. My mother must have stood out. That's where she met my father. From old family pictures, they were a handsome couple, in fashionable western clothes of the 1930's. In one of the photos, my mother reminded me of Ava Gardner, elegant and with long legs, but in Cheongsam (Chinese long dress).

After they got married, my parents settled down in Hong Kong in my grandma's house – a three-storied building with a garden, at the Seven Terraces; ours was named Chee Lan Terrace ('Purple Orchid' Terrace, aka Sands Street). We occupied the ground floor (first floor in American naming) of 33 Chee Lan Terrace. The third floor (second floor in British) was occupied by Grandma. The other floor was rented out. Only the houses in our terrace had gardens. It was perpendicular to five of the other six terraces, with the last one parallel to ours at the east end of these five terraces. Ours had a fairly steep slope that was softened by at least four flights of steps. Going up, the first flight of steps consisted of about 70 steps; the second, third and fourth flights were about 12 steps each and were situated unequally along the rest of the sloping street. In the middle along our street was an open gutter to drain excess rainwater; sometimes it was rushing, other times dry. It was no longer there when we visited Hong Kong with the girls on the same family-history trip in 1989.

I remember one incident that gave everyone a big scare. I must have been ten or eleven years old. We were playing ping pong in my neighbor's garden (ours had a big magnolia tree in the middle plus a couple of smaller trees on both sides, hence no room for a ping-pong table), and the ball flew out into the street. I was chasing it but it went into the gutter. I ran along the gutter that had a sturdy set of steel railings along the whole length on both sides which had been worn smooth over the years by those who needed to hold onto it for support going up or down the street. The water was running fast but I thought I could catch the ball before it reached the top of the long flight of steps to enter the sea. I misjudged the space between the slippery and non-slippery parts of the gutter and jumped over the railing right onto the slippery part that was in the middle. The water carried me down the steps. Fortunately, I somehow landed on my bottom, sliding down the steps as if I were on a water slide, with some slippery plant growth on the steps making the ride soft and smooth. No scratches and no bruises. If I had landed on my side or slipped and fell on my head or elsewhere other than my butt, somehow hitting a wall of the gutter or had a concussion, the water would have carried my inanimate body through the tunnel out to sea because the rushing water at the time would have been strong enough to do so. But it was not my time to leave this world yet. I steadied myself in the less-rushing part of the gutter and climbed out of it. I walked back up dripping wet, scared but unhurt. I remember I did not cry, probably too in shock and scared to. That was only one of the things active boys like me did in those days, but I had to be the one who ended up in the gutter! I gave my family and our neighbors quite a scare because most of them expected me to be swept out to sea. I don't remember that my grandma or mother ever punished me for that.

MY EARLY YEARS

I have no memory of my early pre-war years, especially the first three or four before we left our Hong Kong home to go back to my mother's home village. The only things I remember are two. One is that we had a sliding metal gate (the accordion type) at the entrance to our 3-storied house which was locked at night. The other is one time we had to go to an air-raid shelter a couple of hundred feet down at sea level not too far from our house and another couple of hundred feet from the water front. We all huddled together with other people in a small space. It was dank and dimly lit. We must have gone there at least a few times but I just can't remember clearly. I think the reason may be that, since I have a natural ability to block off unpleasant things, there must be a lot of those in my childhood during the Japanese occupation of Hong Kong. Maybe I had witnessed beheading by Japanese soldiers or seeing human bodies floating on the water near the waterfront, without heads. The cruelty of the Japanese soldiers and beheading at the waterfront were widely rumored after the war. Now, I think there must be some truth to it. Outside of Hong Kong and at my mother's village we never came across any Japanese soldiers until at the end of the war, when some of them were being marched through town by Chinese soldiers.

The trip from Hong Kong to my mother's hometown is a blank. During our 4-year stay in *Wen Lou*, I don't remember much either, except some happy times. The bad times were mostly related back to me by my older sister Yuk Mai (Mai) or Yuk Ling (Ah Sai, aka The Little One, now Lilly). Mai is about two years older than me and Lilly one year younger. When we were children in the village, Mai was our big sister and protector, often fighting with the boys when they bullied me. She bore most of the brunt of any punishment if we were out of line. Lilly and I were totally carefree, as I remember it. We went fishing a lot at a landing with stone steps probably not too far from home because Lilly would run all the way home to tell Grandma or our Amah whenever I caught a fish. We would use earthworm and baited it on a hook Grandma made for me from a needle tied to a thread. We quit that fishing hole after seeing a big snake at the bottom of a dry well next to the landing.

Talking about snakes! One time, a cobra got into the courtyard in our house (must be through the drain) at night and found its way to our chicken coops. There were two or three of them lying on the courtyard where there were a couple of plants growing under the sun shining through the opening in the ceiling during the day. We were all in bed and Grandma heard the chickens sounding disturbed. She told Amah Gui Yung to check out what was happening. Gui Yung went there and patted her hand on the chicken coops to quiet the chickens, and went back to bed. Later, the chickens made noise again. This time, Grandma told Gui Yung to light a candle to look again. When our amah went back with the candle, she saw what had happened, and screamed. The cobra had swallowed a chick and could barely move towards the drain from which it had come. Grandma told Gui Yung to go next door to the village watering hole and ask some of the guys to come and get the snake. Some did and took the cobra away. They were happy to get the snake because they ate the meat and took the snake gall and put it in liquor. This snake gall wine is a tonic known for treating male problems.

On our way home from that fishing hole, we would walk along a stretch of a ditch lined with plants planted there by someone as a fence. There were narrow gaps at ground level among the individual plants. I don't know why I knew or thought there were frogs behind the plant fence. Anyway, using the same fishing line that Grandma made, this time without the hook, I tied a small ball of wet red tissue or crude toilet paper, tinted red, to the thread and dipped it slowly up and down between those gaps. Not too long, a frog would appear, assume a jumping pose, leap and grab it. With a quick and even lift I would land it against my chest or belly, immediately put my left palm over it, securing it there before it had time to escape. Our amah would cook the frogs for us for dinner.

We stayed at our mother's village for four years when I was between four and eight years old. I was a small boy and, because of my absentminded and sometimes clueless nature, a target of bullying for bigger boys. Add to that for being the only kids named Leung among the clan of Ng (*Wu*, Mother's maiden name), we were outsiders. Hence, at school, my sisters and I stood out. Although I don't remember any actual incidents of being bullied, my sisters witnessed them and told me. The only thing I remember is that after school, sometimes Lilly and I would climb up to our roof and teased the big bully walking past our house on his way home, never realizing I would have to meet him at school again. Duh! So, my being bullied was real and my innate ability to block off unpleasant things didn't seem to work well this time. Or maybe it happened so often that this particular repeated occurrence was etched in my memory.

A few other things I can remember vividly: (1) Every end of the semester we would have to find out our class standing by going to a big board next to the classrooms in the playground. The grades and class standings were posted on the board, with the best student on top (No. 1) and the worst at the bottom, such as No. 10 or No. 20, depending on the class size. We could always find our names at the bottom. I don't remember what I had learned at that village school. Nor do I remember any classmates. (2) One day, when the last class was over, we kids had to line up by grade in the playground to be formally dismissed by someone, I guess it might be the principal. I must be 5 or 6 years old and had absolutely no interest even in my teachers or school work, let alone some principal. I have no recollection of what was happening other than I must have been running to the line too fast. Suddenly, my head bumped into the sharp edge of one of the square concrete pillars holding up the school. The impact cut into my left eyebrow near the end next to the left temple. There was blood everywhere. Some adult stopped the bleeding with some fuzzy root of a fern. I don't know how and why it was so handy at the school. A lot of bleeding kids? But later I found out that the hairy root and rhizome of some ferns are well known as being hemostatic (able to stop bleeding). In any case, I was lucky, as there were no complications. I don't remember how long the wound took to heal. But after it did, up to this day, I am still left with a scar along with a dent that I can feel on my left eyebrow, though not easily visible because it is partly covered by the eyebrow hair. (3) My mother once in a while went to meet my father in one of the big cities in China, like *Guangzhou* or Shanghai. I remember once she brought home some shoes for us. She wanted us to put them on to go to school. But we had been already so used to going everywhere barefooted that I couldn't stand the uncomfortable extra burdens. So, I wore them until we were out of her sight and immediately took them off. Then, when we came home, I put them back on before we reached home. My mother must have known what I had done, but I don't recall her ever pointing that out to me. (4) There was a crop failure one year and a famine ensued. I don't remember being really hungry most of the time, because our family had resources, I assume. But I do remember we were fed the precious rice, while adults ate beans. Talking about the village mentality at the time and the villagers' knowledge of nutrition as we now know it! Fortunately, the famine probably didn't last long, because as children we didn't suffer much, except for a fainting incident related to that. One day, on my way home after school, I was hungry and was so weak that I fainted in front of the village temple where the Ngs' ancestor remains were kept. A villager saw me lying on a stone bench in front of the temple and carried me home. (5) Another incident of village life I remember is one time I was helping our amah Gui Yung, pump water to irrigate the rice fields, standing knee-deep in the water. After some time, I suddenly realized my legs had several leeches on them. I tried to pull them out one at a time. But every time I pulled one out, it stuck to my finger. When I used the fingers of the other hand to try to pull it off, it latched onto one of them instead. I couldn't shake any off and didn't know what to do, so I screamed and cried. Gui Yung came and removed them from me. She always took care of things for us as far back as I can remember.

She must have been a teenager during our stay at the village during the Second World War. Back when she was a baby during another earlier famine, her mother could not take care of her. So she came to Grandma and offered her the baby. Grandma gave her some money and promised her she would treat Gui Yung as a part of the family and that when she became of age, she would find her a worthy husband. Grandma did, and Gui Yung was married to our farm-hand, handyman and general caretaker (factotum), whom we called Uncle Yung. I remember they were always part of our family before and after their marriage. Years went by, they had five or more daughters and one son, I believe. The last time I visited them (Uncle Yung long gone) at the village five or six years ago, the son was applying to U.S. colleges to pursue graduate studies in a computer science field and was supposed to be in touch with me. But I haven't heard from him and I don't remember his name other than his surname of Ng and nickname of B Jai (Second Son), the same as mine; but he is the youngest amongst his siblings! They have been part of my family and part of my memory. I hope they are doing well.

Another thing I distinctly remember is one day seeing Japanese soldiers being marched through town and I immediately sensed or knew the war was over and felt joy. Now, I don't know why whenever I think about that or relate it to someone, I feel emotional about it and have to hold back tears.

I don't remember much about my early years in Hong Kong before we went to my Grandma's village to escape the war. But I was happy and carefree in the village, away from the ravages of war, secured under

Grandma's protection. I was happy to see the end of the war maybe because I thought I would see my father again. And not long after that we moved back to Hong Kong. Again, I have no recollection of the journey.

CLUELESS SOR JAI ('IDIOT BOY') TO ACTIVE TEENAGER

Back in Hong Kong, my preteen years from age 8 to age 12 were quite carefree, but maybe sometimes over the limit. I don't remember the details but my sister Lilly later told me that I got into trouble sometimes and Mother would whip me (palms and legs) with a flexible rattan stick. When I retrieved my palm right before the stick would strike it, that made her miss and she was mad. My not crying when she did strike me also made her madder, and that made her hit me harder. It then hurt, and I cried. In those days, corporal punishment like that was common at home and in school. I guess every kid had his or her own way to deal with that in those days. For me, I simply tried to forget about it.

In the beginning, I was pretty much living in my own world, apart from playing with a couple of friends and carousing the neighborhood, playing tricks on some neighbors we didn't like. It was the late 1940's. There were no drugs for kids to get into and our neighborhood was more than a hundred steps above the Hong Kong main traffic. There was a newsstand (or news shed) two gardens down the slope from ours and a convenience store across and over the gutter a short block from the news shed in another terrace perpendicular to ours. The convenience store could be entered from its back door. But to enter from the front, you would have to walk down a flight of steps on our terrace and then up another longer flight leading to that terrace. The store was on the ground floor of its first building. So, when I was sent there to buy things sometimes, I always took the short cut, entering the store at the backdoor. Even that might only be at most 100 feet or so from our garden, I sometimes would get distracted on my way and forgot about what I was supposed to get. I had to go back and ask. It might take me a couple of times on occasion, but I always accomplished my mission, at least as far as I can remember. Grandma and Mother never made a big deal out of this when it happened; and they continued to send me out on those errands. Probably because of this and other absentminded things I used to do, my father called me "Sor Jai" (*shazi*) sometimes, but not meaning it. In Cantonese, depending on the tone and the person who uses it, "Sor Jai" can be a casual endearing term for a spacey kid like me or to mean a stupid boy; it is also used to mean a mentally handicapped child with obvious symptoms. I am sure my father had not used it to mean I was stupid because he was a person who bragged a lot, about himself and his children whenever they excelled in something. And I had a lot for him to brag about while I was growing up, which I always hated and swore I'd never do that to my children. Then, after I have become a father and grandfather, I can't help but brag a little about them, because I am so proud of them. As to bragging about myself, I have refrained from doing so even after living in my adopted country for 56 years, observing some of my fellow Americans padding their resumes and indulging in exaggerating their accomplishments. Now, I am no longer shocked when I see people 'marketing' themselves and their products by using exaggerations and sometimes downright lies. It is really sad to be like that. My impression of this unique American trait is that sometimes, when an American knows 10% of a subject, there is a good chance he would talk and behave as if he were an expert. Unfortunately, in recent years, lying is trending to become the new 'normal' among many American politicians and businessmen.

SCHOOL WAS NOT MY THING UNTIL...

I never liked school but somehow, I managed to progress from one level to the next without paying much attention to what I was learning in general. When I was interested in a subject, I would excel in it, but with subjects I didn't like or considered boring, I just managed to get a passing grade with not too much effort. It's the same with social situations. When I am obliged to be in conversations that are boring I simply tune out, but if unsuccessful, I'd keep very quiet with my mind drifting in and out and not getting the gist of the conversation. I have been caught many times when someone tries to bring me back into a boring conversation and I have no idea what it is about, this makes me seem really dumb in some social encounters. Who would want to socialize with someone who seems deaf and dumb and doesn't know how to make small talk? More than once or twice, a new acquaintance would just walk away and avoid me thereafter. At first I thought it was discrimination, but now I know it might have been my absent-minded or 'clueless' nature.

I went through the Hong Kong school system from elementary school through high school before going to college, in a rather unconventional manner. A few things stand out in my memory.

In first grade, I was once detained after school because I wrote my name consisting of three characters on an exercise book which occupied the whole cover. Seeing that I was late coming home, my mother or Grandma was worried and sent my sister Mai to fetch me. At the time I had no idea why I was detained just for writing my name big, since nobody told me to write it certain ways. Or was it that I had tuned out and didn't hear what the teacher told us? Today, psychoanalysts would have a field day with analyzing my psyche.

Then, when I was around ten or eleven, I attended elementary school in the Chinese section of St. Louis School run by Salesian priests and brothers. I was expelled for not paying attention in class. When my mother went to beg the prefect (priest in charge) to take me back, she was told that I couldn't sit still and talked too much in class, thus disturbing other children. I remember him distinctly because he was tall, big and had a big belly. Kids were scared of him. I can still visualize him every time I think about him. He used to walk among the children on the playgrounds during recess from the English section to the Chinese section, with his cassock blowing in the breeze. One time, I was surprised to see him actually watch me and another student practice ping pong as we were both on some varsity team at the high school section. That was after I had returned to the English section and had become a 'normal' student after being expelled a couple of years earlier and he had refused to take me back.

During that year in 'exile' from St Louis, my parents sent me to another school up on a hill, called Chung Cheng Middle School, named after Chiang Kai-Shek (aka Chiang Chung Cheng). Chiang was the general who was the last leader of the Republic of China before the Chinese Communists drove him to the island of Taiwan in 1949 and established the People's Republic of China in the mainland. The school was no longer a walking distance from home and I assume I had to take a bus every day to get there, though I have no recollection of the bus rides. Also, I have no idea why I attended that particular school. Being well connected to some high-level politicians in the Kuomintang Party, my father must have known some of the people who founded that school and pulled some strings to place me there. I remember at least once, probably twice, the granddaughter of Dr. Sun Yat-sen visited our home in Hong Kong for whatever reason. I was twelve or thirteen years old then, and learned that Dr. Sun was the founder of the new Republic of China after having successfully overthrown the Qing Dynasty. I am sure I had learned it repeatedly before, but it never sank in until then. I was very impressed and that connection was etched in my memory.

In addition, the year 1953 was Queen Elizabeth's coronation and there was some sort of arts competition among Hong Kong school children. Paintings and drawings by students were being judged and some selected to be sent to England for exhibition. One of my paintings (a portrait of Dr. Sun Yat-Sen) was among those selected to go to England. I have no idea where it ended up.

Scholarship-wise, the year I spent at Chung Cheng Middle School is mostly a blank. However, I do vividly remember lunch breaks and a couple of teachers. Since the school was half way up the hill, we climbed the hill picking berries and throwing stones at one another. There were usually four of us. We had fun until one time, and the last, one boy got hit on the head and was bleeding. That scared us and we never did that again. I don't recall whether the injured boy got treated or how we got away with explaining that to our teachers or school administrators. Also, I don't remember any of the boys' names and what they looked like. However, I do remember two of my teachers at that school, our gym teacher and our English teacher. Our gym teacher was a short, stocky man with bulging muscles and was good with pommel horse and rings. He used to strut around near the equipment and showed off his skill, especially while girl students were around. Our English teacher was a well-dressed lady on high heels who used to sit on her chair sideways at one side of her desk with her legs crossed. Since I was sitting in the front row, I used to stare at one of her beautiful legs showing through the slit of her 'cheongsam' (body-fitting Chinese dress with slits on both sides along the legs). I must have been in my hormone phase then, and started noticing the opposite sex, because I can still clearly remember her face, slightly buck-toothed, but beautiful.

THE ENGLISH LANGUAGE STARTED MY SERIOUS QUEST FOR KNOWLEDGE

During the year when I was attending the Chung Cheng Middle School with fun-filled lunch breaks while they lasted, my parents hired an English tutor for me. She was a chubby Chinese girl in another Terrace (To Li Terrace) perpendicular to ours who was maybe three years older than me and a student at a well-known English girl's school run by Maryknoll nuns. She was a good teacher. Finally, I seemed to have found my calling and I picked up English fast and was at ease with it. For some reason, I felt like a new door to the world had been opened to me. And I actually enjoyed reading English books on my own. It seemed I had struggled all my life (all thirteen years of it) with the Chinese language and finally it was great to find something that came easily for me and learning was fun. I guess I was never meant to be a Chinese scholar, or for that matter, any type of scholar that requires memorizing things. And to think of it, I can't even quote, not to mention recite, a single poem in Chinese or English despite the fact I must have learned at least some English ones in high school. Then in college, I used to like reading English poetry, though no further than just reading.

In any case, instead of struggling with Chinese that was (and is) difficult for me, learning the English language gave me a new life. Perhaps my brain is wired differently than other Chinese. I found a whole different world out there that I could explore with much more ease. That feeling was similar to what I had experienced when switching from skiing to snowboarding when I was in my mid-sixties, never to go back to skiing again. I could ski okay as long as the slope was not crowded because I couldn't turn gracefully as good skiers like my daughters do. I need more room and fewer skiers in my path! That made skiing not that much fun. But with snowboarding, after you have fallen enough times on your head and shoulders, you finally become comfortable with it and you are king of the mountain! I envy young people riding and jumping on the slopes so gracefully and they seem to have so much fun. Although I have paid my dues on the icy slopes of Mont-Tremblant in Quebec to become a medium-level rider, at my age, I am satisfied with just being able to cruise and turn down the slopes. After I finally moved to Colorado six years ago, riding on powder is a whole new experience. In the first three years, I had just learned enough to handle powder of less than a foot, when a car accident incapacitated my snowboarding – some young woman hit me from behind at a stop light totaling my Volvo XC-70 (but still drivable) and her SUV (Tahoe) needed to be towed. For three years now, I haven't gone back to the slopes, and I miss riding. But I probably wouldn't do it again even after this accident is settled. Then again, who knows?

MY HIGH SCHOOL AND COLLEGE YEARS

After my year at Chung Cheng Middle School, I passed the entrance exam to the English section of St. Louis School (about a mile from home) and now I was on my way to be a good, and eager student! Life was much simpler in the 1950's, no computer databases to cross check 'trouble-makers' like me. The English section might have no idea that I was expelled only a year earlier from the Chinese section. Yet I recognized the same prefect who refused to take me back when my mother pleaded.

I loved my new English school at St. Louis where all the instructions were in English, except Chinese subjects. My favorite subjects were the sciences (biology, chemistry, physics, math, and geography) and of course, English too. Right from the beginning, I found myself in the A class, out of classes A, B, C and D, with A being the best academically, each up to 45 students. I excelled in all science subjects and math. Then, after one summer break during which I read 30-35 abridged versions of English classics by authors like Charles Dickens, Sir Arthur Conan Doyle, Jane Austen, H.G. Wells, and many more, I went back to school and found myself excelling in English as well. However, reading so many books, sometimes late into the night on dim light, ruined my eyesight. I could no longer see from the back row where I used to sit with a couple of my buddies (one of whom is now my brother-in-law, Anthony Fung Yee-Wing), and had to be moved to the front. Soon, I had to start wearing glasses.

Although that summer of intensive reading had ruined my eyesight, it made me one of the best in English 'overnight' in my grade from Form 1 to Form 2 (comparable to Grade 8 to Grade 9). During my last year (Form 3) at St. Louis, I was selected along with a classmate called Tong Yuen-Yao to represent our school at the Hong Kong Catholic Schools/Students' Press Club, or something like that, as I can't remember the exact name; nor can I remember what magazine or newspaper they published. Tong was consistently the Number 1 student at our class, while I was somewhere between 2 and 10 or a little further down there, because some boring subjects dragged my overall grades down. Last time I heard, probably twenty-five years ago, he was married to a Quebecoise and was a professor in Quebec somewhere.

Around that time, I think my grandfather had already come home from Havana, living with his third wife and daughter in Kowloon. Every second day of Chinese New Year, I used to take a live chicken (a capon, I believe) along with some other goodies in a big shopping bag to Grandfather to wish him Happy New Year and to collect lucky red envelopes (with money) from him for myself and my sisters. The trip must have taken most of the day because I remember I had to walk down to sea level from our home, take a bus or the street car (tram) to Hong Kong Star Ferry, cross to Kowloon by ferry, take a bus in Kowloon to near where my grandfather lived and then walked to his apartment. Hong Kong in the early 1950's was quiet compared to now and much safer for kids to move around without an adult.

My grandfather had left much of his business in Cuba for his young cousins to manage before he came home. There was talk at home for me to go to Cuba to learn and take over his business. An exotic place like Cuba fascinated me. So, on my own, I bought a copy of "Teach Yourself Spanish" of the "Teach Yourself..." series published in England, and taught myself Spanish. I did all the exercises in the book and finished it probably in months. It seemed to come naturally to me; and with something I liked, I had no problem concentrating. At that time, I had an excellent memory with English and Spanish, and I was probably the best speller in English at school. But now, I probably rank average among the general population. I am one of those people who never can learn a language by listening and then speak it. I have to learn a language by sight and grammar, with speaking only after I have learned the basics. I admire people who can listen and repeat the sentences without learning basic grammar. Anyway, by the time I flunked out of St. Louis School, I was able to read and write Spanish, though I had no chance to converse seriously with anyone until I was in college. Then, I met Padre Marcelino Andreu at the National Taiwan University (NTU) in Taipei in 1956-57, who then became my mentor during my college years.

After I had taught myself Spanish, I was on a roll. The two other languages that I taught myself (at least in the beginning) are French and German, just to read, not to write, both before I graduated from high school and left for Taiwan in 1956. These languages came in handy later in college and graduate school. During my graduate studies, I passed both during one year without having to take any courses. Translating from a page or two of technical German and French into English was easy for me as you were allowed to use a dictionary. I guess I did quite well with German; it prompted my examiner to write "Excellent piece of work!" on the slip of paper announcing "pass" or "fail" results after the language exams.

In the 1950's and 60's, most PhD programs required reading ability of two foreign languages and the University of Michigan was no exception. However, for whatever reason, Spanish didn't count at Michigan, maybe at other universities too. In any case, when I was in NTU, I took courses in French and German among students of the Department of Foreign Languages. French was taught by a Quebecois priest from Canada, and was rather easy for me, since I already knew Spanish and had self-taught myself to read French. But the only thing I remember about that class is that during the final exam, it took me maybe only half the time to finish and hand it in, to the stares and admiration of my fellow students most of whom were from the Foreign Languages Department. That must be one of the very few times I felt on top of the world in something without working hard at it. Maybe also English at the National Taiwan University.

As English was a compulsory subject so that students could at least read English books and journals, all of us had to take it as a freshman. I remember my teacher was an older lady in her fifties. Early on, she must have noticed that I looked out the window a lot, and decided to talk to me in English after a class, and found out that I had an English education in high school. So she gave me permission to skip her classes. But being brought up to respect elders, I tried to make extra efforts to attend some of her classes and tried to pay attention whenever I was in class. But that was hard! I was finally excused and officially exempted from taking English and was granted full credits.

During the first two years in college, I seemed to have a lot of free time because I skipped classes a lot, mostly language and civic types of classes. There was one class called "Three People's Principles." It was a politics or Chinese constitution class and I couldn't understand a word the professor said because his Mandarin (*Putonghua*) was very thick with some accent (Sichuanese or Shanghainese). I figured there was no point to sit in class, falling asleep anyway. And since it was a big class and I didn't think the professor would miss me, I arranged with a couple of my classmates to lend me their notes for me to copy afterwards. Throughout my college years, I had a group of classmates (my core support group) who were very good to me. They included Howard Hou Hong-Kee (nicknamed Monkey because he was very skinny, actually wiry, with no fat in his body) who was also my roommate among eight (in the general campus) or six (later in the medical campus) of us. Monkey was not from a privileged family, so he didn't own a bicycle. During our second year in Pharmacy, we still lived in the dorm on main campus but we had to take a couple of classes in the Medical campus that was maybe fifteen minutes away by bike. He used to ride sideways in the front on the main frame of my Hercules bike to attend those classes. At that time we never even gave that a second thought about our safety, because it seemed like a lot of people were doing it. After graduation, he became a pharmacist practicing his profession in Vancouver, Canada, all his life. The last few times I met with him when I had to visit Vancouver on grant research business between 2000 and 2005, he was still working full-time.

Monkey is one of the most persevering persons I know. He studied very hard but some of the most important subjects he would receive just a passing grade. No matter, he succeeded in finishing four years of Pharmacy school and has dutifully practiced his profession all his life. I think of him a lot whenever I look at a picture a friend (Don Scott from Glen

Rock, N.J., I believe) gave me 40 years ago which depicts a frog half-way being swallowed by a heron but the frog has its hands around the bird's neck preventing itself from going down the bird's throat; and the caption says, "Don't ever give up!" That reminds me of Monkey's perseverance! During our four years of Pharmacy training, he was my lab partner in different subjects. After he became a Canadian pharmacist, he raised a family, and became a very good skier.

My other classmates include Kwok Hong-Nin, a pharmacist in Hong Kong, by now must be retired; Nancy Ying-Chee Lee (nee Ma) used to own a small biotech firm but also maybe retired now; and Georgiana Siao-Ju Hou (nee Liu), who is a retired California pharmacist. Without their support, I would not have made it through college with the non-technical subjects. I am forever in their debt. Once in a blue moon, I still have nightmares about sitting at an exam of a subject I didn't like and about which I didn't know much. I am so relieved when I wake up to know it is only a dream! I detest boring tests!

Cutting classes allowed me to have free time to go to my favorite coffee house in downtown Taipei where they always played classical music, not just excerpts or selected movements, but often serious music like the whole symphonies, quartets or concertos. Even though I had a record player and a sizable collection of records, I couldn't enjoy music in a room with seven other roommates. The coffee house was perfect for me. My favorites at the time were Beethoven's Ninth (the Choral) and his Violin Concerto. I used to follow the German text when the chorus was singing the Choral in his Ninth because I had a copy of Schiller's poem that came with the set of Beethoven's symphonies that I had bought in high school. At the young age of nineteen, I actually could understand what they were singing and I used to lose myself in the music. The clientele of the coffee shop was mostly students, but never more than a dozen or so at a time when I was there. There seemed to be a silent agreement to only do your own thing and no talking. I met a fellow student from my class there a few times. Can't remember his name now (Yan something) but he was a top student and one of the few native Taiwanese students with whom I sometimes socialized. He didn't seem to have any particular close friends. Or maybe he was like me who just wanted to be alone, reading or studying while listening to classical music.

I graduated from high school in the year 1956, not from St. Louis School but from Literary College, a new English high school started a few years earlier. After I had flunked three or four subjects in Form 3 (equivalent to sophomore year here), I was expelled from St. Louis. I don't remember exactly the names of the subjects I had flunked, but they had to do with Chinese (Chinese history, dictation, or composition?) and with memorizing things. However, I distinctly remember one of the subjects was music for which my teacher gave me a 59 (60 being the passing grade). That must have been on purpose. Maybe I was a trouble-maker in his class. If so, I don't think I would have intended to be. I can't recall, though I still remember his name, Siu Leung, Siu being his surname. And I'll never forget the final music exam. We had to sing a Steven Foster song standing in front of our classmates. Some of them couldn't carry a tune and the scene was quite comical, trying not to laugh. I was in the school choir (bass) and I was at least not tone deaf. But I never finished my song after a few tries, because I couldn't help laughing, looking at my classmates (especially my buddies) making funny faces at me. My story would have been quite different if I had not flunked music but stayed at St. Louis to graduate with my classmates and followed a more conventional route.

After my expulsion, I decided to skip the junior year and attend my senior year at another school so as to finish school sooner. Since I knew I was good at English and the sciences, I could skip Form 4 and go directly to Form 5 (senior class). So, I took the entrance exam to Literary College and did so well that the English teacher asked me after I had finished his part of the exams where I studied before. I said "self-study," and he didn't pursue further. This was probably the way teachers dealt with potential incoming students who were too embarrassed to tell the truth that they might have flunked out of a better school. Later I found out I was the first student of that school with the proficiency in English that he had not seen before. He was a good teacher, and was the first one who helped me simplify my sentence structure and acquire a simpler writing style. My sentences used to be long, at times up to half-a-page, though grammatically correct. Reading too many English classics (including unabridged ones) must have exerted a big influence. Now, I always try to be conscientious in making my sentence structure simple, even though I may not always succeed.

My final year of high school at Literary College was originally meant as a conduit of sorts for me to finish high school and then see what would come next. In those days in Hong Kong, all high-school students had to take the uniform School Certificate Examinations. If you passed, you showed you had scholastic skills to go on to college or take up certain jobs, like one as a clerk in civil service with job security. There were minimal requirements for types of topics one must pass. It would have to include English (dictation, compositions, etc.), at least a subject in science, and one in civics (like social studies here). I passed the bare minimum of 5 subjects with 4 credits which meant that my grades in those 4 subjects were at the top 1/3 of all students having taken the same tests. I was told I could have gotten a distinction in English (top 3.3%) if I had not made 2 mistakes in the dictation test. One of which was the word "innumerable" that our English teacher had mispronounced as 'innumberable.' Anyway, I was an excellent speller then. Now, I have lost it, and have to depend on spell-check, which is not that reliable. Literary College was so proud of my results that it displayed my grades (the 4 credits) prominently behind the entrance to the school. I have no idea if the school still exists. Regardless, with that school certificate verifying I had graduated, I was able to pursue my studies in Taiwan. At the time, our family finances were deplorable. I think besides pawning my parents' valuables, at one time we even took in renters (a nice looking couple with a little girl maybe six or seven years old). They took the smaller of the two rooms on the main area next to the living and dining rooms. It's hard to imagine how we all managed with two families and one bathroom. I am now so spoiled!

My father was an entrepreneur. So income was not steady during that period. But he insisted on me going to college, not just getting a civil service job as many of my fellow graduates did. Uncle Siu came to my rescue. [see **Chapter 3: Uncle Siu & Aunt Pauline...**] He was going to support my college studies by sending me U.S. $10 a month. At first, I intended to study medicine as my first choice but my grades didn't meet the standards for medicine of the NTU and I was assigned to Geology. My first year in NTU majoring in geology was interesting and noneventful. I loved geology and the field work. I could have gotten a degree in this field if I had a choice, but I didn't. My family insisted that I get an education in a field that was employable. So I tried to get into medicine again the following year and retook the entrance exams to NTU after my geology year. This time my grades were still not good enough for medicine and I was assigned to pharmacy.

Now, looking back, I am glad I studied Pharmacy and not medicine. Otherwise, my physician job would have been so engrossed with patients and drug therapy that I would never have had the time and extra mental energy with mental clarity to have discovered that the so-called scientific drug therapy is nothing but the budding stage of a modern version of herbal therapy (esp. traditional Chinese herbal medicine), starting to gather true human experience only after a new drug is approved. With traditional Chinese medicine, it already has over 3,500 years of documented clinical experience, whereas modern drug therapy only has a maximum of decades of human experience, yet instances of side-effects turning into new diseases have already occurred which require new toxic drugs to treat; and the vicious cycle goes on. [see **Chapter 12: What's Wrong with Drugs…**]

At pharmacy school, although the lectures were all in Mandarin (*Putonghua*), we used mostly American textbooks so I had no problem studying. We had many of the same general science textbooks used by students in the U.S., like Linus Pauling's Textbook of General Chemistry. Since I could never take notes, especially in Chinese, I just jotted down some highlights (words and phrases) of professors' lectures and later studied the English textbooks. I wrote the exams in English after asking the respective professors' permission and none of them objected. With some Chinese subjects, like one civic/political subject and another dealing with military training, my classmates, knowing my handicap, were very kind in lending me their notebooks to copy. This also applied to some technical subjects for which there were no English textbooks. Without my classmates' help, I probably would not have gotten a BS in Pharmacy from NTU with an average overall grade of B but an A in pharmacognosy, which had allowed me to apply to graduate schools in the US.

I believe in fate, que sera, sera! I have been mostly lucky all my life. I tried to plan maybe a few times, but things never turned out as planned, so I made lemonade whenever I was dealt a lemon. And it helped to have a network of classmates/friends who understood at least my handicap of not being able to listen and write at the same time while in college and then later, a loving and competent wife who is smart and organized.

TO GRADUATE SCHOOL IN AMERICA!

For my graduate studies, I only applied to two universities, the University of Washington and the University of Michigan. Michigan offered me a teaching assistantship sight unseen, probably based on my English test (at that time administered by the University of Michigan). I got a 97% in the test that included writing an essay on some topic assigned on the spot, conversation (for maybe 3-5 minutes), and also some reading comprehension test, but I am not sure.

I was plain lucky to be able to go to college and then graduate school. The University of Hong Kong was very expensive and there was no chance I would go there. Since my chances of going to Cuba to learn my grandfather's business were also nil because the Cuban revolution was brewing, the only choice for my higher education was to go to Taiwan. That was at the insistence of my father, even though we really had no steady income from Cuba anymore. That was when Uncle Siu stepped in to help out. He supported my five college years in Taiwan by sending me 10 USD per month which was sufficient for all college fees (education, housing, and books, among others) with extra for weekend entertainments (e.g., coffee house, movies, concerts, eating out, & snacking). [see **Chapter 3: Uncle Siu & Aunt Pauline ...**]

Around that time, in the mid-1950's, many high school graduates in Hong Kong went back to China for college because it was the only place they could afford. Uncle Sam was well aware of that. So, it subsidized Taiwan (Republic of China at the time) in building special overseas student dormitories for mostly non-Taiwanese Chinese students from Hong Kong and other parts of Asia. Its closing one eye to pirate printing of American textbooks and many other types of books also helped students' finances a lot because pirate-printed books were everywhere at a tiny fraction of regular prices. Taiwan was the only island territory the Kuomintang had, the rest of China being called The People's Republic of China was held by the Communists. One of my paternal aunts and her husband (a senator in the Taiwanese government) and a couple of children lived in Taipei. I think she was number 11 among my father's siblings while he was son number 9. Also, an 'uncle' (Uncle Doon) connected to my Grandma's village (*Wenlou*) was in Taiwan, after retreating from the Mainland to Taiwan with Chiang Kai-Shek. He was a colonel in the Chinese air force fighting the Japanese alongside the Flying Tigers (volunteer American air corps in China formed by General Claire Chennault) during World War II. He was the son of the other native son of the village who made his fortune in the U.S. and a peer of my Grandfather who went to Cuba. Each had a classroom named after them side-by-side at the local school. Uncle Doon ran away from home and joined the Chinese Air Force. He had been with it all his life. When I was in Taipei attending NTU, he was a colonel. For the first couple of years when I lived on the main campus, my dormitory (#13, built with American subsidies) was not far from his home, and he used to pick me up on weekends in his government-issued jeep to have dinner with his wife ('Auntie') and his three preteen to early-teen boys. Auntie was an excellent cook and I thoroughly enjoyed her cooking. I remember helping at least the older boy with his English and that Uncle Doon was very good and stern with the boys and that he treated me very well, like family. However, after the first two years on main campus, my life and studies got busier. Visits with Uncle Doon and family became less often and eventually we drifted apart. Since I graduated from NTU and returned to Hong Kong, I have not seen them again. This is one of the many things I did or didn't do that I still regret.

It was maybe the second or third year when I was in Taiwan that I found out my cousin (Yuk-Chang) from my Seventh Uncle before he went to England for his college education was in Taiwan. He was working as a coal miner around Taipei somewhere. I only visited him once. I remember I had to take a bus to get to where he was, perhaps an hour's ride, I am not sure. A day before my trip, it had rained around the mines and there was mud on the hill. I had to hike up the hill in the mud to get to his little hut among others. They must have belonged to the mining company. All I remember is he had a wooden bed consisted of a few planks with a crude straw tatami on it as mattress. Maybe there was also a chair or some table for holding things, as the floor was muddy and not paved. It was dim inside. I felt so badly for him but I couldn't do anything. Also, he looked unhealthy. Not long after my visit, I learned from my father that he had died from some miner's disease.

Looking back at my childhood-to-college years in Asia, I feel very lucky under those circumstances. I somehow ended up finishing high school and college and was going to start a new life in America. First, being admitted to the graduate school of the University of Michigan was not easy with academic records of barely a B-average like mine. And then, being offered a teaching assistantship sight unseen was to me like a miracle. I didn't realize how lucky I was at the time, but I do now. Without the financial support of Uncle Siu and Auntie Pauline, I would not have gone to college, period, let alone finished it with a Bachelor of Science degree in Pharmacy. And without the teaching assistantship from Michigan, I would not have become a pharmacognosist, specializing in herbal medicine, writing to you today, trying to tell you and the world about what is wrong with our drugs and 'herbal' supplements. They can be made much better if we start doing something about them, especially by resetting our priorities towards the less fortunate by forgoing at least part of the excessive profits.

CHAPTER 2

People Who Helped Shape My Character While Growing Up

When it comes to a person's character, I believe heredity and childhood background play the most important roles. I was born with a unique set of personal characteristics, different from any of my siblings. If I were born today, I would probably be considered a person with attention deficit hyperactive disorder (ADHD) and most likely managed by pharmaceuticals, contributing to the financial enrichment of Big Pharma & Company. Thank heavens my family didn't drug me!

Since childhood, I have always been easily distracted but full of energy and can't sit still for things of no interest to me, even now at my advanced age. When I am not interested in something (like gossip or matters of no concern to me) and if I am obliged to be present, I simply tune myself out. My family must have known this, yet as far as I can remember, they never pointed out my deficiencies. Instead, they overlooked them. They tolerated me until I left home for college at age 18! Whenever I think about that, I am so grateful to my family for loving and nurturing me the way they did, especially Grandma and my amah (Ah Shun) when I was a child. I don't remember much of my mother during my preteen years and my father was seldom home during that period.

Despite my handicaps (especially during my preteen years) I grew up pretty much like most active boys. I participated in all kinds of sports, like ping pong, football (here in America we call it soccer), basketball, and later, tennis. I was on our high school varsity basketball and ping pong teams. And with subjects like English, science, and other languages in which I had intense interest, I could focus and work on them with no problems for long periods of time. In my sophomore year before I flunked out of St. Louis High School, I was one of the two students representing our school in the Catholic schools' press club in Hong Kong, though I don't remember its exact name. [see **Chapter 1: Growing up in Asia**]

I made friends and played like most other kids. However, because of my basically shy nature, making friends did not come easily for me in elementary school. Someone else had to break the ice, the rest was then easier because of my easy-going, non-meddling nature. Nevertheless, I don't remember any of my friends in elementary school that I made before I became a teenager.

In high school, I seemed to have no difficulty making friends. As I did well in the English section of St. Louis School, both academically and in sports, I quickly became among the 'elite' of the Class A students. There were 4 classes in each grade, from A to D, with each class composed of 40 to 45 students. The classes were arranged based on academic standing, with top students in Class A and less academically proficient students in Classes B, C, and D. There were six grades in high school: Form 1 to Form 6. In Hong Kong, Form 1 was considered high school, but it was more like our Grade 8 here. Form 5 was the graduating grade. After that, the highest grade, Form 6, was only for students planning to attend the only university in Hong Kong - the University of Hong Kong, or some British university in the United Kingdom. In any case, if you passed the School Certificate Examinations at the end of Form 5, many countries, including the United States and Taiwan, would recognize that as a high school diploma that would allow you to apply to attend college or university.

Starting from Form 1, I had always been ranked within the top ten students in my class of 45 which was basically among 180 students in my grade. During one semester in Form 2, I was actually ranked number 2 in my class, which was the highest I had ever achieved academically, though at the time I never thought much about that. The next year, when I was in Form 3 (sophomore), due to financial troubles and family discord at home, I flunked out of St. Louis. Then, I skipped Form 4, went to another school (new and freshly accredited), and finished my final year there, passing the School Certificate Exams with honors that qualified me as having officially finished high school; and I was a year ahead of my former classmates at St. Louis.

The people, other than my family, who had shaped my character from childhood up through college, include the following. Since some were contemporaries with one another, my narrative of them may go briskly back and forth.

WONG WAN-YEUNG (YEUNG BUDDY)

It was in the first of my four years in high school from Form 1 to Form 5 (skipping Form 4) that I first met Wong Wan-Yeung, nicknamed Yeung Tsai or Yeung Buddy (YB). I was about 13. He was about three years older than me. I never found out when he was born or exactly how old he was; or maybe because those numbers weren't important to me, I simply forgot about them even if he might have told me. In those days in Hong Kong, while some families might celebrate birthdays of their children as we do here in America with birthday cake and presents, my family's tradition for celebrating kids' birthdays was to simply give the birthday boy or girl a hard-boiled egg in its shell, dyed red. I never found out why a red egg, but that was the usual way I found out when it was my birthday. But that doesn't necessarily mean I was one year older. In Chinese custom, you become one year older on Chinese New Year's Day. To further confuse finding out the real age of anyone around that time, I started learning Western customs of celebrating the Western New Year. That made birthdays that much less memorable or important. Seriously, a spacey kid like me would actually care to keep track of these things!? Only when I was a grownup, especially when our first child, Amy, was born, did birthdays start to mean something.

Nevertheless, as far as I remember, YB was like a big brother to me. Now, I try to remember how I met him, but I simply can't. Since I don't keep a diary or any detailed written records, I have no way to find out.

In my childhood until I left home for college in Taiwan, I lived in 33 Chee Lan Terrace (aka Sands Street) except for a few years when the Japanese occupied Hong Kong. Then we went back to China to live in my mother's ancestral home in the village of *Wenlou, Xinhui* county for four years, when I was between four and eight, and returned after the Japanese were defeated. The Hong Kong house belonged to my maternal grandmother. It was in a rather exclusive neighborhood called the Seven Terraces consisting of our terrace (Chee Lan Terrace) half way up the hill on the west side, running down to sea level on a slope. Another one (Li Po Lung Terrace) on the east side parallel to ours also ran down on a slope to sea level but it was much narrower and without any drainage gutter. The other 5 terraces were perpendicular to ours and Li Po Lung Terrace with stairs running into both streets (terraces). Our street was the widest and had a water drainage gutter several feet wide running down the middle. The gutter was surrounded by well-worn steel railings that ran all the way down to sea level a few hundred feet long. At sea level, there was the general Hong Kong traffic, though at the time when I was growing up, it was nothing compared to what it is now. [see **Chapter 1: Growing up in Asia**]

Our life at the Seven Terraces was quite sheltered, mostly separated from the hustle and bustle of the city. As children, we moved around freely among the terraces, particularly the three or four terraces closest to our house, three-quarters up our terrace. They all had stairs heading down towards our terrace, also known as Sands Street. I don't know why, as there was never any sand around our neighborhood, unless it was named after someone with the name of Sands. The highest terrace was Hok Si Terrace now called Academic Terrace. The next highest was To Li Terrace, followed by Ching Lin Terrace, Hee Wong Terrace, and finally the lowest one, Tai Pak Terrace, named after a famous Chinese poet (*Li Bai* aka *Li Tai-Bai*) of the Tang Dynasty who lived during the 8th century.

As described earlier, our street was quite steep. No one would try to ride a bike on it (unless it's mountain bike, fast forward to the present, like in America). To ride any bike, you would have to first carry it from the street at sea level up 70 steps, ride 50 or 60 feet, carry it for another roughly 12 steps, and ride another 20 feet to my house.

Yeung Buddy lived in the highest, Hok Si Terrace. My house was only 4 houses from his terrace plus 2 flights of steps (each of around 12 steps) and then half-way up his terrace. His terrace now no longer exists; in its place are a couple of big high-rise buildings without entry from our terrace.

His family lived on the third floor. It took just a few minutes to walk from my house to his. When I had to look for him, I just called his name in my loudest voice and he would respond by appearing on the balcony. If after a few calls and he didn't show up, I knew he was not home. Evidently, loud calling was common in those days. None of my family ever told me it was inappropriate. Often, when dinner time approached and I was missing, my grandma, who had a solid loud voice, would call my name from our window. I could hear her from Yeung Buddy's neighborhood and other friends' gardens on our street and the woods behind it. If I didn't hear it, someone who heard it would tell me. Of all the years I knew YB, I remember I actually knocked at his door only once for sure, maybe twice. One thing I remember is the staircase leading to his front door on the third floor (second floor in British naming) was very dim. Being brought up in a couple of traditional old houses and having been often scared quiet by amahs and maids when little, I had my share of ghost stories and I didn't like dim places.

Since YB was as shy as me, it was fate that we somehow met. We were best friends all through my high school years and most of college years. Between his terrace and mine, there were two flights of steps of about 12 steps each separated by a flat area that served as a bridge over the water drainage gutter. The flight of steps on my side of the gutter ended in the flat area next to the woods. The drainage gutter continued along the back of YB's terrace all the way up beyond the Pok Fu Lam Road to a reservoir further up the hill. The railings continued all the way up to Pok Fu Lam Road. YB and I used to sit on the railing in the flat area facing the sea at night when everything around us was dead quiet. There were only occasional pedestrians walking from sea-level a couple of hundred feet up towards us. Most of the time, they went home to their own, lower terraces. Rarely would anyone walk past us to the highest terrace where YB lived. Sometimes the view of the sea was spectacular, with an occasional ship, such as a freighter, ocean liner, or junk passing our view. We would sit there on the railings for hours on end from dusk till dark during many evenings with our toes or instep anchoring us by a lower rung of the railings, so that we wouldn't slip into the gutter when feeling too comfortable. We both dreamed about faraway lands. He dreamed about being a scientist like Einstein and I dreamed about being a doctor or herbalist helping people like my grandma and great grandfather, the village doctor. Another one of my heroes was Albert Schweitzer. For a year, I taught myself Spanish and we talked about my going to Cuba to learn and take over my grandfather's business and build a lab as Edison did to do experiments in chemistry. He wanted to go to America. I lost hope of going to Cuba when my grandfather's business was facing loss with the inevitably approaching Cuban revolution.

Yeung Buddy and I both liked classical music and we both admired Albert Einstein. I was rather mature for my age after having done my share of things that annoyed others, like neighbors. So when I met YB in my early teens, I had already found my focus, mainly languages, sciences, and math. I had other younger friends but, by then, I found them sometimes still doing silly things that didn't interest me anymore. I remember at home my grandma and mother used to start referring me as acting like an old man. YB and I talked about everything or just sat on the railing above the water drainage watching the ships go by and the few people wearily coming up the steps and the slope, spending the rest of their energy to make it home from work to the Seven Terraces. For some reason, we just felt comfortable with each other, sometimes we talked and other times we just sat, not obliged to say anything. From many of these occasions, I found out YB had probably a troubled childhood. He had both parents. He was the oldest, with two younger sisters. They all appeared normal to me, but we were never formally introduced. Once in a while I met them on the street and simply exchanged acknowledgements such as a nod of the head or a smile, but never talked. In fact, I never exchanged any words with his sisters. He never talked about his family, or about girls. YB never had a girlfriend but was always interested in my talking about girls. Just about the time we started to be close friends, maybe when I was 14 or 15 years old, I started noticing girls. But none seemed to interest me except Mary Chow Pui-Ying.

MARY CHOW

Mary had a slightly older sister. I don't remember her name. Yeung Buddy was interested in her, but like me he never did anything. We always referred to them as Big Choice and Small Choice, meaning older Choice and younger Choice because we didn't know their names except of all the girls in our neighborhood they were our choices. They were both beautiful with very fair and smooth skin and nice smiles (at least Mary's because I never had the occasion to see Big Choice smile).

Three things about our 'relationship' stood out which were difficult to forget. The sisters lived with their parents and a younger brother on To Li Terrace, the terrace immediately below Yeung Buddy's. They occupied the second floor (i.e., first floor by British counting) of a house there. The rear window of their home was facing YB's first floor (or ground floor) at street level right at the beginning of a long flight of steps, maybe 50-60, leading to a flat section that constituted the rest of Hok Si Terrace before another set of stairs leading to Pok Fu Lam Road. I am sure when Mary was home she would have heard me calling YB when I visited him. When I was attending St. Louis High School, I used to take the Pok Fu Lam Road that winds around a mile or so, at up to a hundred feet above sea level, past much of the campus of the University of Hong Kong to get to my school. Before I got to Pok Foo Lam Road I had to walk past Mary's rear window and the rest of YB's terrace. On coming home from school I would take the same route in reverse. This happened for a year or more until I flunked out of St. Louis and attended the last year of high school at Literary College which required taking a bus of 30 to 40 minutes at sea-level. But when I was still going to St. Louis, on my way to and from school, I always looked at Mary's window. Once in a while, I saw her there looking out, and it made my heart pound. And I always wondered if she noticed me. That was in high school. I don't remember how I went to the same school during elementary school before I was expelled. And all that was before I had any inkling there were girls other than my sisters in this world.

The second memorable thing was that from the front window of our house I could see Mary's front balcony past a couple of tree trunks in our garden. It happened that that window was facing the left side of the long flight of stairs coming down Mary's Terrace. From that window, looking past the top of the steps, I could see the balconies of some of the houses, including Mary's. Incidentally, my English tutor (the chubby girl) in an earlier year, lived a few houses closer to our terrace but her house was out of view. [see **Chapter 1: Growing up in Asia**] But Mary's balcony was quite far, one couldn't see it too well unless one used binoculars. But that was my secret, no one but YB knew at that time. So, I never used binoculars. However, I could see anyone walking down the steps clearly once he/she approached the lower steps, including Mary and her sister. And Mary usually glanced over at my window after she turned right from the steps to head down the slope on our street.

The third thing I found unforgettable was one of our household helpers somehow ended up working for Mary's family. It must be after the Cuban revolution finally started to affect my grandfather's business in Havana and the money from Cuba was drying up. We could no longer afford domestic help. I remember I had to go to the pawn shop several times to pawn my father's and mother's jewelry, including one time my father's Rolex watch. I can still remember the pawn shop clearly. It was at sea level, about half way from my home to the closest cinema we used to go to, maybe about a mile away. The pawn shop's entrance had a tall solid wooden screen situated at a few feet right after you crossed the doorway, actually a threshold, about a foot high. The wooden screen covered the whole front door. So, after you walked around this heavy screen to the other side of the room, there was room to do business with complete privacy. Nobody could see you from the street. Inside, there was a wall with metal bars between it and the ceiling. A small window was in the middle of those thick bars where you had to reach up to give whatever objects you wanted to pawn to the man sitting up looking down at you in his imposing and intimidating perch. I remember after my transactions, I would make sure to count my money and put it in my safest pocket before I would quickly exit the place so that nobody would see me. If I lost the money or somebody picked my pocket, we probably wouldn't have money for food for days or weeks.

About the same time, I finished Form 3 (sophomore) and was sixteen or seventeen years old. I flunked three or more minor subjects and was thrown out of St. Louis. To go to the new school I had to take a 30- to

40-minute bus ride. I sometimes wondered if Mary had asked our maid about me and my family. It was tough to be a teenage boy at that age, especially when I was so insecure about girls. Both my sisters, Mai and Lilly, were beautiful girls. Mai is two years older and Lilly one year younger. They got all the attention because I was just a boy, not handsome or spectacular, mostly living in my own world. I never thought of girls until I noticed Mary. At that age I felt I was ugly because I was used to being the least attractive one in the family; and I had heard family conversations that basically confirmed my feeling. I didn't outgrow that sentiment until I was in college when most of my female classmates were very nice to me; and I knew if I had asked, they would have gone out with me. Actually, one of them followed me to the U.S., but I have no idea where she ended up. She was a nice and pretty girl. It's just that I had no romantic interest in her. I feel badly about that. I think she finally married some guy from the medical school. I hope they have been doing well.

During my Form 5 year of high school, I bumped into Mary on the bus many times because we were going the same direction out and back. She smiled at me and I did the same, but never had the courage to talk to her and she was always by herself! And on 2 occasions, YB and I went to the cinema at sea level about 20 minutes' walk from home to see movies featuring classical music. One was "A Song to Remember" with Cornel Wilde playing Chopin, I think. Or maybe it was the "Great Waltz." Not quite sure. The other was "Rhapsody" about a violinist and a pianist with Elizabeth Taylor being the star. I still remember the music they played included excerpts from the Violin Concerto of Tchaikovsky and the Second Piano Concerto by Rachmaninoff. When we came out of the theater, we bumped into Mary, by herself one time and with a girlfriend another. She smiled at us, but I did nothing other than smiled back. What a dumb fool! On second thought, at my 'old-man' phase at the young age of 15-16 per my grandma and mother, I might be thinking of our family finances. I was the boy of our family and eventually would be responsible for it. I knew deep down in my heart I could not afford financially and emotionally to get involved in real dating and love. So, I was a chicken.

After I graduated from high-school, both YB and I decided to go to the university in Taiwan. He was already in a technical college in Hong Kong. But he wanted to major in electrical engineering and get a university degree. He passed the entrance exam to the same university I had applied. He got his first choice, electrical engineering. But I did not get to study medicine and was assigned to geology. The main reason was after skipping Form 4 (Junior year), I lagged behind in math and that part of my entrance-exam grade dragged my overall grade down. So, YB and I both went to National Taiwan University in Taipei. We also got assigned to the same dormitory room, all eight of us. It was dormitory 13, Room 301.

When I was in Taiwan, I finally had the courage to contact Little Choice (because I didn't know Mary's name yet) long distance. On looking back, I was a real chicken. But how to contact her? At the time, I had at least her address. With only an address and without a name, I addressed the envelope to "The Younger Daughter" or something like that in English and wrote her in English, because she went to an English School run by Maryknoll Sisters. I don't remember what I wrote but I think I did mention I had met her various times on the Terraces and on the bus. I never expected the letter to be answered and I was just hoping. But some weeks or maybe months later, she did write back. During my years in Taiwan, we corresponded steadily many times. It was purely platonic love. Nobody knew except YB in the beginning. However, when I returned to Hong Kong during Summer Holidays, I never had the courage to visit her.

But my first and only platonic love kept me out of trouble, particularly unnecessary girl trouble, all through my college years. Even though I had many chances with girls, I was not interested in any of them; though I considered Georgiana Liu and Nancy Ma very good friends who were also two of my core supporters in letting me copy their lecture notes. Some of my classmates knew I had a girlfriend, but none knew the truth. That had kept me focused on my studies as well as allowed me to have my peace of mind to read all kinds of books (philosophy, psychology, music composers, poetry, and self-help, you name it) while improving both my written and spoken Spanish with Padre Andreu as well as improving my reading skills in French and German. Now looking back, I feel lucky to have Mary as my platonic love that had put me on the right path of focusing on getting a degree.

Finally, after my graduation, I returned to Hong Kong and taught chemistry at the Salesian School on the opposite side of the island as St. Louis School. In the meantime, I applied to graduate studies in Pharmacognosy and was offered a teaching assistantship by the University of Michigan. I left Hong Kong the summer of 1962. Shortly before I went to the United States, I learned about the premature death of YB in Canada from the man who had been a fixture (at his shed) on our block selling newspapers and miscellaneous items. This man had seven daughters and finally had a son. He told me YB had died from some sort of cancer. I had no other details of his death. The last time I saw YB was when my roommates and I went with him to the Taipei Airport to see him off to Canada to attend McGill University in August, 1958.

When I was in the United States, Mary and I continued to exchange letters. One time when she went to Japan on vacation, she sent me pictures. Other times she also sent me pictures with a couple of close friends together. I urged her to come here. But she couldn't for whatever reason. When I returned to Hong Kong in 1965 for the first time to visit my family, I finally got the courage to call her to meet me at a coffee shop near where she lived. But instead, she wanted to meet me at her home. So I did. But it was rather awkward. Even though we were alone in her living room, our conversation could be heard easily in adjacent rooms in the house. Mary was pretty much what I had expected. She was not slim, nor overweight, maybe 5 feet 2, and was soft spoken. I don't remember a thing of what we talked about. But somehow I felt uneasy. I don't remember whether we planned on meeting again, or whether or not I had asked her out. Most likely I had forgotten to ask her out. In any case, I think our meeting was no more than 30 minutes. Again, that might be wrong, trying to recall after all these years – more than 53!

After I left Mary that day, that was the first, and also the last, time I was ever 'alone' with her in person. And life moved on. Although we had corresponded several more times in another couple of years, my memory of our relationship got fuzzier and fuzzier. As I was finishing my Ph.D. studies, I was thinking of settling down. Also, I was finally tired of my platonic-love phase. After I got my Ph.D. and accepted a postdoctoral position with Dr. Einar Brochmann-Hanssen, Professor of Pharmaceutical Chemistry at the University of California Medical Center in San Francisco, to San Francisco I went in the fall of 1967. Within months, I met Barbara Haas through computer dating (in the period when computers were still the size of a whole room using punch cards), fell in love, and I never looked back. Barbara and I married the next fall (1968). We have 2 lovely and talented daughters, Amy and Camille, with very different personal characteristics. Amy takes after me in her absent-mindedness and creativity and Camille takes after me in her meticulousness in writing. Amy's daughter (our granddaughter) has inherited a whole mix of genes from both our sides as well as her dad's. She definitely got her mom's and my energy and creativity genes as well as her grandma's organization abilities. She also got some of her smart genes from all of us, including her father, a computer scientist. I like to show people a picture of her, saying beforehand that she looks exactly like me, and observe their puzzled reaction to see a blond kid with no Asian features, except perhaps a little in her eyes.

Although the relationship between Mary and me didn't work out, her love (expressed a couple of times in her letters to me during my college years), along with Yeung Buddy's, and Padre Andreu's friendship and mentorship during my teenage and college years, kept me out of trouble. All that allowed me to concentrate on the tortuous path that started at home and ended up what I am – a pharmacognosist and jack of all trades.

DAVID MOK

David and I went back a long way, starting in St. Louis High School at the English section. We were in the same grade, though I don't recall which class he was in. Class A or B, or other? He must have also flunked out of St. Louis, but a year earlier than I did, and also skipped a grade. We both ended up in the same Form 5 class of about thirty students in Literary College. That class was like a bunch of misfits with painful histories to hide, who went to that school using it only as a shortcut to graduation. A few were from well-known Catholic schools like St. Louis but I don't remember their names. Usually, students from these schools would not switch to an unknown school like Literary College, unless under extraordinary circumstances like mine or David's, whatever theirs might be. I must have known these at the time but forgot about them over the years because they were not important for our friendship. The school was accredited only a couple of years earlier and thus officially allowed to participate in the Hong Kong school-certificate examinations. Once you pass the exams and get the certificate (we used to call it 'School Cert'), you have officially finished high school. A diploma from any high school would not be worth as much as a school cert. When I met David there, I recognized him and we became close friends right away.

David was skinnier and a little taller than I was. He was soft-spoken, like YB, and also shy. It's funny, my best friends have been mostly quiet, with one exception, Fong Chuen-yen, who used to swear a lot (see the section on him). David was from a broken family. His father lived in the Philippines and occasionally sent him money. I know that because, when David received money from his father, though rarely (maybe a couple of times a year), he would spend it like there were no tomorrow. He would splurge on Western restaurant meals and on entertainment, including records, movies, and shared his enjoyment of it with friends. And I was one of the very few, if not the only one, with whom he socialized. I would go with him to eat Western food, even though I preferred my Chinese favorites that he also liked. He lived with his mother and a sister in the eastern part of Hong Kong, near the school. For me, it would take about 30 minutes of streetcar ride to get there. I met his mother only once. But I remember her as being like a businesswoman, dressed elegantly, and not like most women I knew in those days. She seemed to be genuinely happy to meet one of David's classmates. David, like Yeung Buddy, seldom talked about his family. Come to think of it, most of my good friends are private persons. None of them gossip and most of them are introverts, including Jaime Dajer of the Dominican Republic whom I met more than 35 years ago.

David received a monthly allowance from his mother, but I don't know how much. He was a generous soul and I guess he didn't keep track of his money well. Sometimes he actually went around hungry. When I first noticed that, I started to treat him to our favorites of wonton noodle soup and beef with gristles sold at street-food stalls and in some cafes that offered them. And during those times, I also started bringing him home for dinner. My grandma and mother treated him like one of us; so did my other family members, and he was well liked. After dinner, I would ride with him back to his area in east-central Hong Kong. We would hang around in Causeway Bay area until late. At the time, Yeung Buddy was still my best friend and big brother. However, since my daily school commute was now at least two times longer, he and I had less time to sit on the gutter railings to chat. By then, Mary and her family had moved to Causeway Bay and I somehow knew where she was because perhaps our former household help had told me, though I don't know how. By that time, I had let David into my secret, but not all of it. Because of my family's finances, I simply couldn't get into a romance and dating situation to detract from my education. In any case, Mary's big window looked over the Causeway Bay area, with people milling around, and there were benches, like in a park. Mary lived on the third floor, or maybe the fourth; can't remember. Many times, late at night, we saw her looking down but I didn't know if she was just looking. David and I spent our Form-5 year going to Causeway Bay at night a lot. David also decided to go to the university in Taiwan. He selected engineering and was assigned to Tainan in southern Taiwan.

In college, he came up to Taipei most holidays and stayed in our room because one of our roommates was a native Taiwanese, Wu Ju-Dun, who would go home to Taichung (Middle Taiwan) on holidays. I only recently learned from one of his daughters that Ju-Dun had passed. She sent me a memorial video of Ju-Dun at the urging of her mother. Ju-Dun was a very gentle man and I am glad to know he left such a big and loving family. I wish them all the best.

For two years or so, I was a private tutor of English to two sisters and their brother, all high school students. They were pretty girls. I got that job from my aunt whose husband was a legislator and he recommended me to his fellow legislator (or some rich businessman) who was the father of my students. I introduced the second daughter to David and they dated. Consequently, I was happy to see David in Taipei during holidays, because by then, YB had already gone to Canada. The summer of 1959, he stayed in my bunk all the time when I was back home in Hong Kong on holiday. I think he had a good time dating my student. I have never found out how that ended. Anyway, friends from childhood are special because we have gone through so much together and know one another so well. Despite the fact we hardly ever write one another, when we meet years later, we pick up where we left off as if we saw one another only yesterday. After I left for the States in 1962, I went back to Hong Kong for the first time in 1965. After that, I started to go back around the mid-1980's with Herbalife's founder Mark Hughes, Dick Marconi, and Michael Moers, taking them to visit different academic institutes, herbal factories, and historic sites. [see **Chapter 6: Herbalife**...] During the 1980's and 2000's, I met David various times. By then, I was married and had children. David was also married, to a Taiwanese woman, but not to my student. He spent his time between Hong Kong and Taiwan. He was not in his engineering profession, but appeared to do well in real estate, with houses in Taiwan and in Hong Kong besides the ones in which they lived. Later, I heard he decided to live permanently in Taiwan and moved back to Taiwan. Last time when I saw him in Hong Kong, he had gained weight and looked healthy and happy. That must have been over ten years ago. I think he is one year older than me, so he is up there in years. I hope he is alive and well. I miss his steady and quiet friendship!

FONG CHUEN-YEN

As he has no Christian name, we always call him Ah Fong or simply Fong as long as I have known him. I don't know his family background. Fong is about my height, same build. Another quiet guy but could be animated like me among friends. We were in the same graduating Form 5 class of misfits, at Literary College, when we met, along with David and Anthony Sze.

I don't know much of Ah Fong's pre-Literary-College life except he was known among friends as a martial arts (gong fu) expert. From what he has told me and what I have gathered from mutual friends, he learned gong fu when he was a kid. By the time I met him in high school, he was already an expert. But I have never seen him practice. Also, being a real expert, he never flaunted it and you would never know looking at him, just a nice quiet guy. I had watched him demonstrate a few moves only once in our dormitory in NTU to a few friends and roommates. I could actually hear and feel the air movement several feet away from him. It was just like the fake sound of gong fu movements in movies. However, that was only sound effect; the sound of Fong's gong fu movement was real.

For whatever reason, he was also planning to go to Taiwan to attend NTU. His chosen field was electrical engineering, same as YB's. And he got assigned to the same university and dormitory as mine. While YB and I were in Room 301 at Dormitory 13, Fong was in the room at the other end of our floor with seven other students who were Pui Ching graduates. Their room number was 311. For a long time, I thought Fong was also from Pui Ching, a Chinese high school as well-known as St. Louis. I learned to know all his roommates and sometimes hung out with them there. When Fong was with his friends, he used to swear a lot. Talking about swearing, no other language or dialect I know, or am aware of, has more swearing words and phrases than Cantonese. I myself don't swear in Cantonese or English but I had maybe one or two other friends who did. But none is like Fong. Even so, he doesn't swear in front of women and families.

Fong and I didn't socialize too much in Taiwan as he had a Taiwanese girlfriend, I believe. After he graduated and returned to Hong Kong, he immediately found a job as manager of manufacturing with the American company, Lockheed Corporation, in charge of some sort of manufacturing there. Through his work, he came to know a lot of important people. Like me, he is an entrepreneur at heart. So, he has been involved in various companies. During this time he and his wife have raised a family with 3 children who now all have technical careers in the States. With the career as an entrepreneur, you win some and lose some. Or, as my friend and fellow indexer and abstractor, Ed Tello (with the NLM), used to say, "you win some and lose a lot." Since Fong lost his last electronics company through his partner's fraudulent participation, he was running someone else's company in Guangdong for a few years, commuting daily between Hong Kong and *Dong Guan* in Guangdong. When I was in Hong Kong three years ago, he was the same Fong. We talked on the phone but he could not come to have dinner with me and another good friend, Sin Lam-Kwong. He was happy working, the way he has always been. And he is my age or even a year or 2 older! When he had a chance, he would be still making deals. I totally understand his situation. The day you tell an entrepreneur to stop working or to count beans, you may as well send him to his grave. During my most recent visit to Hong Kong in January this year, he was fighting cancer. He had gone through chemotherapy and was taking some Chinese herbs. He looked good. I hope he can hang in there.

Starting around the mid-1980's, with a hiatus of a few years after the Tiananmen revolt, I had been going to Hong Kong and Mainland China at least once every year, sometimes up to three or four times, until 2014. Most of the years, Fong would meet me at the airport in Hong Kong when I arrived, usually in the evening. After checking into the Sheraton or, in later years, into one of the Marco Polo hotels, we would go to eat my favorite noodle dishes. We would carry on as always, no formalities. I hope to see him again during my next trip.

ANTHONY SZE

I met Anthony or more commonly known to us as Ah Zee or simply Zee at Literary College. Zee was a couple of years older than I. He was a big muscular guy, maybe around 5 feet 10 inches tall. He had a hearty laugh. I had no idea (or had forgotten) where he used to study. But his intention was like that of most of us – pass the School Certificate Exams and then see what lies ahead.

Once in a while, he used to join David and me to hang out together. I used to help him with his English and sciences. When I first met him, he already had a little boy maybe two years old. He and his wife and child lived on the second floor (first floor) of one of the houses lining the street (I think Queen's Road) near the Central region of Hong Kong about half way between Star Ferry area and the Seven Terraces. He was a very hard worker but English didn't seem to come easily for him. So, he tried to make up by working twice as hard as others. Unfortunately, even with that, he didn't pass the School Certificate Exams because of his English. That must be very hard for him. I can't remember what he did then because I was busy preparing during the summer of 1956 to go to Taiwan that fall for college, along with my buddies Yeung Buddy and David. All I know is he had to repeat Form 5 and finally passed the School Cert and got a civil service job with Immigration. During my college years I at least went back to Hong Kong during the summers maybe three times. David, Zee and I would meet for dim sum or some noodles in Central. But I don't remember if he was an immigration officer during my college years. I do remember I saw his son when he was an older boy maybe five or six, and said to myself that he was such a handsome and bright kid.

We seldom wrote each other, if ever. Just like with my other friends. Then, at least twenty years later, I started to go back to Hong Kong and China regularly on business in the 1980's. During one of those earlier trips, as I was approaching Immigration check point, I saw an inspector observing people heading towards the lines at check point. He seemed to recognize me and walked towards me. Then when we made eye contact I recognized him. He put on some weight but not fat or overweight. He simply led me through Immigration to the front so I didn't have to wait in line. He was in full official uniform, very impressive, especially on a big guy. I couldn't tell his rank but I think he must be pretty high level because he seemed to be in charge.

In any case, during my one to three times a year visits to Hong Kong during the 1980's, I bumped into Zee several times at Immigration during arrival and he would notice me and escorted me past the long line. I remember we would plan to meet for noodles in some café after I checked into the hotel and he got off work. Whenever I was in Hong Kong, my friends never let me pay the bills. It was no different with Zee. They all knew I like simple food, noodles, noodles and noodles; no fancy or expensive dishes! As he and I were always busy when we met on those occasions, most of the times a simple meal was all we could spend the time for. So I never met his boy and family after he grew up.

I always wonder how his son is doing, especially after the several times I had seen him, Zee just disappeared. Later, it was Fong or David who told me Zee had died. I don't know of what.

MARCELINO ANDREU, S.J. (PADRE ANDREU)

Most of my childhood education was at St. Louis School run by priests of the Salesian order. My family started me first in the Chinese elementary section and later in the English high-school section. But none of the priests there converted me, though I was liked by the key priests in that school, including Fr. Alexander Smith from England and Fr. Alexander Machuy (Fr. Ma) from Mexico. Father Ma later became the principal of Salesian School and hired me as soon as I graduated from college as its chemistry teacher during my last year in Hong Kong. There was also Fr. Groot from Holland, my English teacher who was also in charge of my class (like what we in the US would call my home-room teacher); he was with my class for two years. However, it took Father Marcelino Andreu (I called him Padre Andreu) to convert me to Catholicism when I was in Taiwan at college. As far as I could see when growing up with the Salesians and later with the Jesuits, neither was in-your-face type of missionaries. They seemed to be dedicated to education first and then religion would be up to the students. I remember we always had a class of catechism but I paid little attention to it. There were a couple of overtly devout Catholics among my classmates who used to hang around the priests a lot but they were not among my buddies; though some of my buddies were also Catholics. Later I learned that religion is very personal. Only God (under whatever name) and you know what is in your heart. I can compare it to patriotism now in America. You can't just say you are patriotic and wave an American flag to show others that you are, while at the same time your actions are to subvert our democratic ideals for personal gain.

I met Padre Andreu (P. Andreu) at the Catholic Student Center in Taipei where the main campus of NTU was located. He was a Castilian Jesuit from Spain who spoke Castilian (Castellano), the Spanish I taught myself in high school. I guess it was rather unusual for him to see a Chinese freshman at college who had taught himself to read and write Spanish but never had seriously spoken it. Maybe due to curiosity he was interested in me and took me under his wing. He spoke to me in Castilian whenever we were alone and he thought appropriate, and corrected my writings as well as answered my questions whenever I had difficulty with some tough words or sentences, including slang. At the age of 18 to 21, I soaked up whatever he taught me. My meetings with him had been at least several times every month for three years, first when I was a freshman in geology and then as a freshman and sophomore in pharmacy. I might have also seen him once in a while after I had already moved to the medical school campus, and probably more often in my senior year because I was taking two semesters of French on the main campus at the Foreign Languages Department. But I don't remember much of all that despite the fact that after I had been baptized a Catholic, I used to go to mass regularly at the little chapel at the Catholic Students Center on the main campus, as I remember. As befitting my clueless nature and selective memory, I tended to block off unimportant or unpleasant events and recall only those that stood out. So, later when I felt disillusioned with organized religions, I considered many religious events unimportant and tried to erase them from my memory, which is why it is so difficult for me now to recall what amounted to daily routines during the time when I was in Taipei with P. Andreu. My disillusion with, and retreating from, organized religions took many years to happen.

After I returned to Hong Kong and then settled in my newly adopted country, the United States, I continued to go to mass. For many years, I had been supporting Boys Town by sending it checks whenever I sent money home to my mother out of my teaching assistantship's stipend and later from my salary or income from consulting. Then, years into my marriage, when our first child Amy was about four years old, a New York Times article on Boys Town's finances was published. It seemed Boys Town raised so much money over the years that it didn't know what to do with it. After I read that story, I figured it had so much money that it wouldn't need mine. So I sent that money home instead. Since then, reports of sexual abuses by priests appeared all over the world and have kept appearing. All these prompted me to reassess organized religions. I was disappointed in the Catholic Church, even though growing up with the Salesians, I had nothing but positive experiences; same with P. Andreu and the Jesuits. But then I had also read about some so-called Christians in my adopted country, especially some father-to-son types of inherited enterprises, amassing mega millions for themselves in the name of Christ. Yet they may only give token pittances to charity so as to qualify as non-profit organizations, enriching themselves while at the same time, spreading hatred instead of true Christian love and values. They even supported liars and exploiters of the poor and the sick. Now, I feel disillusioned and I hesitate supporting any Christian group. However, I still believe in the basic teachings of the Christian faith, and of Buddhism, as well as those of ancient philosophies based on love and charity as lived by my grandma and amah.

That reminded me of my growing up with Grandma and, to some extent, with my amah. Grandma had lived her life the Buddhist and family way. Starting when I was a child, I observed that Grandma always treated others with compassion and kindness. She was physically small, barely 5 feet tall, but had a loud voice. She also had a big heart. I started to learn my family's ethics and morals by observing her actions. Also, I learned them from my father's side through my grandfather's teachings as my father has related to us. Family tradition and ethics were important in China. When I was eight or so, after we had returned from China after the Second World War, until when I was probably twelve or thirteen, we almost always had someone (relative or otherwise) from China living with us who had nowhere to go during tough times. They included 'cousins,' 'uncles,' 'aunts,' and anybody remotely connected to us. Most of them were from *Wenlou* (my mother's village) but some from *Huizhou*, my father's home town. I seldom paid attention to them because I lived in my own world around that age. Nevertheless, I remember at least two because they stayed with us for months if not a year or two, at different times.

One was my cousin, Leung Yuk-Chang, the oldest son of Seventh Uncle, before he left for England and then Malaya. [see **Chapter 1: Growing up in Asia**] We used to call him "Chang Gor" or "Older Brother Chang." He must have lived with us a long time during my preteen years, because I remember he was the first one ever to help me with my English. Other than that, I don't remember much about him. Later, when I was a college student in Taiwan, I saw him again before he died not long after.

The other person who lived in our house in Hong Kong was a nephew of my father's, though not from his Fifth Brother. He was of my father's age or perhaps even older. He used to be a colonel in the Chinese army before the communists drove Chiang Kai-Shak to Taiwan. He was really tall, over 6 feet, and skinny. I don't know why he stayed with us or where he went afterwards. The only thing I remember about him is he might have been a drinker but at that time I had no idea what that meant because none of my immediate family drank. He used to keep a small bottle of something (now judging by the shape of the bottle - flat and about an inch thick – I believe it might be whiskey) in the cabinet under the staircase going to Grandma's floor upstairs. I saw him drink from it. There was never a lock to that cabinet. I don't think I had any idea what that was. I was around ten years old and I was curious. Perhaps I thought it was some yummy juice. One day I found myself near that cabinet with nobody around. I took the bottle out, opened it, and hurriedly took a gulp of it. Boy! I thought I was going to gag and die! I hadn't taken just a sip like you would try to taste something. I must have taken in half a shot! Since I had drunk it in such a hurry, I couldn't even spit it out because it was down my throat already, burning all the way down to my stomach. I never went near that cabinet again. I wonder if that experience has prevented me from drinking later in my life. Even though I am not a drinker, sometimes I had to toast a little on business. This burning sensation from my mouth all the way down my stomach was later experienced again when I had to toast with *mao tai* in the 1980's at some business dinners in China. *Mao tai* is the strong liquor made from sorghum which Premier Chou En-Lai used to toast President Richard Nixon when he first visited China in 1972. I can say my experience with it was like drinking a strong liquor and burping gasoline for hours afterwards. Though my cousin's drink did not give me gasoline burps as far as I remember.

When I was in Taipei with P. Andreu during my college years from 1956 to 1961, I really didn't know that much about his personal background. All I knew was that he was a Castilian Jesuit from Spain and lived at the

Catholic Student Center where there were rooms for priests and nuns to hold language classes. If I remember correctly, there was also a small chapel attached. But I always met alone with him in a small room with a table and chairs for up to four people. Sometimes I accompanied him on errands. He was easy to converse with; and he used to call me Alberto. We talked about everything, family, traditions, philosophies, religions, and psychology, you name it. At that time, especially my first three years in Taiwan, I was an avid reader. I read everything I could get my hands on, including English literary classics, poetry, self-help, philosophies, psychology, music composers, and other subjects. I found P. Andreu to be an open-minded, compassionate, and trustworthy person. He soon became my mentor. We also discussed religion and faith. For a long time I was trying to understand faith through the eyes of a scientific-minded young man, looking for proof. But that didn't get me too far. I finally realized that one must believe and have faith. Without that, you don't have a religion. Certain things are not provable. It's between you and God (or whatever name and religion you call this entity). It's personal. P. Andreu showed me by living it his pious way. I never knew that his family lived it all their lives as guided by his mother until only weeks ago when I tried to search the Internet on information about him. As a start, I Googled him in Spanish "Padre Marcelino Andreu y estudiantes Taiwan." I thought that would have enough key words to draw the appropriate information on him from the Internet. What showed up on my laptop screen shocked me. First listed was on the "Andreu family and Garabandal" in Spanish. Then, immediately following was "Ecela Student: Albert Leung..." in English. After my initial shock, I began to realize I did go to the Ecela Escuela in Santiago, Chile, for a 2-week Spanish conversation immersion course. Not long after, at the school's request, I sent them a review (in Spanish) of why I had wanted to go there and what my experience had been. The school's translation is basically correct except that, although I might have had learned Spanish in Hong Kong first, I now live in the United States and had gone to Santiago from here, and not from Hong Kong.

After finishing college, I didn't keep up with my spoken Spanish for years, apart from some brief exchanges of greetings with Spanish-speaking friends or colleagues. Since I am not the kind of person who is good with small talk when trying to make friends in English, I find it difficult to do so in Spanish also. Though I tried to keep up for some years in the past few decades during my travels on long plane rides by reading Spanish newspapers instead of my usual spy or action English novels. I used to pick up a copy of *El Pais,* a newspaper from Spain, during transit at Schiphol Airport in Amsterdam every time I travelled to Europe. Later, I switched from English novels to *El Pais* and an Argentinian newspaper, *La Nacion,* that I subscribed on my Kindle. That lasted many years. Then, starting more recently, maybe three or four years ago, I started to set my cell phone in Spanish and read the news in Spanish. When I am tired of the Spanish news, I switch back to English to read the news in English. They are always different. This helps me to get back and retain much of the Spanish I had learned when I was a teenager. But now, if I don't know a word, instead of only consulting the dictionary once when I was young, it usually takes me two or three times encountering it before I can remember its meaning. Three years ago, for whatever reason, I thought I could brush up my spoken Spanish in a couple of weeks in an immersion course. But I was wrong! After decades without hearing Spanish spoken regularly, I was more rusty in listening than anything else, especially in Chile. Only after I had returned from Chile was I told a couple of times that down there they are the fastest Spanish speakers!

In any case, if I had not gone to Santiago, Chile, for a Spanish immersion course at Ecela Escuela and written a review at its request, I would never have been 'connected' to P. Marcelino Andreu and his family.

Here is what I've found out about P. Andreu and his family, by searching him on the Internet. His mother had six sons, four of whom became Jesuit priests – Alejandro, Ramon, Luis, and Marcelino. Alejandro was in Venezuela, Marcelino in Taiwan, and Ramon in Central America and the United States. P. Luis remained in Spain because the Jesuits didn't want to let all her Jesuit sons go abroad as missionaries while leaving her alone at home. So they let P. Luis stay in Spain to be near her. P. Marcelino was the youngest and P. Luis was a couple of years older.

After I got my BS Pharmacy degree in 1961 and left Taiwan to return to Hong Kong that summer, with no clue what was happening to P. Marcelino Andreu and his family. I went about my business teaching and preparing to go to the United States for graduate studies. [see **Chapter 4: Adulthood in America**] I didn't keep up with P. Andreu except maybe writing to tell him I was going to America when I was ready to leave Hong Kong the following year. So, I had absolutely no idea so much had happened to the Andreu family during all the years since I left Taiwan after my graduation until I decided only very recently to find out more about him and started to search the Internet. The reason is that since he was my mentor when I was studying in NTU, I wanted to say something about him out of gratitude. But after all these years, especially after my disappointment with organized religions, I remember so little about him and me together. So, after searching the Internet I have found out that he was from a very devout family and that they were part of a 'miracle' at a small village called Garabandal (San Sebastian de Garabandal) in northern Spain.

During the summer of 1961, while I was preparing to teach chemistry at the Salesian School in Hong Kong that fall after I had returned from Taiwan, there were visions and ecstasy experienced by four preteen girls there, starting in late June and early July. They attracted a lot of attention, including that of P. Marcelino Andreu's brother, P. Luis Andreu. On his first visit, P. Luis was not sure in the beginning, but after observing the girls in ecstasy closely he knew something profound was happening. He went back on August 8, 1961 for the second time, and again observed the girls in ecstasy. Then, eyewitnesses saw him become tense and heard him utter the word "miracle" four times with tears in his eyes. On his drive home with friends early next morning, he died peacefully after saying his last words, "This is the happiest day of my life."

Since then, the Garabandal story has been spreading worldwide.

If you simply type the word "Garabandal" on Google, you'll see websites with the story of the girls in ecstasy along with images or videos. Both P. Luis Andreu and P. Marcelino Andreu can be seen in one of the videos in an American website in English. I recognize P. Marcelino there, though he was not identified or mentioned. This was real and amazing, which eventually could be another well-known miracle site such as the Lourdes in France, even though the promised Garabandal miracle has not yet occurred. What are the chances of my being mentored by the brother of a priest involved in a miracle?!

There seems to be too many coincidences. I went to a Catholic school, (St. Louis) as a child, and got expelled twice from the same school run by Salesian priests. In college, I met my mentor, P. Marcelino Andreu, a Jesuit. Back home in Hong Kong, I taught Chemistry for a year in Salesian School run by the same priests. Then, almost 58 years after having spoken Spanish with P. Marcelino Andreu for the last time, I felt I should speak Spanish again, and decided to go to Chile for an immersion course. In a review of the school, I happened to mention my Spanish-language experience in Taiwan with P. Marcelino Andreu. After that, I thought that would be the end of my Spanish experience until I finally was about to finish my memoir. I wanted to tell my readers about the people who had a positive influence on my character while I was growing up. I included P. Andreu even though I was already an adult when I first met him, because he had a major role in helping me build my character during my college years. Just like Yeung Buddy being my Big Brother when I was in my early teens, P. Andreu was my mentor in college in my late teens and early twenties. I had already written something about him earlier, but when I reread it, it was rather skimpy. That was when I started to search him on the Worldwide Web and discovered all the information on him and his family; and the information on my last Spanish experience was on the first page together with that of P. Andreu's family.

Not long after P. Luis death, their mother (then 65 years old) entered the cloister of the Salesian (Salesa) Order at the Visitation Convent in San Sebastian, Spain, and became Sister Luisa Maria. I also found out P. Marcelino Andreu was born in 1927 and passed in 1998. He was about 30 years old when I became his student in 1956/1957. He later became the Director of the Catholic Student Center in Taipei.

Whatever all these coincidences may mean, I feel privileged to have been a student of P. Marcelino Andreu's and to have been mentored by him, as well as to have spoken Spanish with him during much of my college years. I am honored to have my name appearing together with the Andreu's name when Googling P. Marcelino Andreu along with student and Taiwan. As I said in the chapter **Growing up in Asia,** I believe in fate: Que sera, sera!

My passion is to save traditional Chinese medicine and to start modernizing it the right way so that we can produce time-tested natural medicines to afford the sick and poor an alternative to the current expensive, toxic drugs and potentially toxic chemical supplements. Helping the less fortunate is not only the Christian thing to do, it is also the basis of all religions and any decent family's tradition.

CHAPTER 3

Uncle Siu and Aunt Pauline — My College Education

Uncle Siu and Aunt Pauline were part of my life growing up in Hong Kong after World War II and our return from my Grandma's home town, *Wenlou*. Before that, I was too young to remember anything other than the metal accordion gate at the entrance to our house and a nearby air-raid shelter. The prewar part of Uncle Siu's story was mostly from what I have learned from my family. Although I have seen pictures taken at the wedding of Uncle and Aunt, where Mai, Lilly, and I were all dressed up in our best, I don't remember much about them before my preteen years. At the time, I must have been around eight or nine. It was probably a year or two later that I started to love Aunt Pauline. She was beautiful, gentle, and had a very warm smile.

As I was growing up, she always made me feel loved and treated me as if I were her own oldest son. Uncle Siu treated me the same. Their boys, Raymond and Daniel, in turn, looked up to me as if I were their older brother, because I was roughly ten years older and I loved them. When I was a teenager staying with them during holidays or over long weekends, when the boys didn't do their homework or misbehaved, Aunt Pauline was quite stern with them. She didn't hesitate to use the rattan stick just as my mother used it on me. Education was a top priority to Uncle and Aunt.

Our house in Hong Kong at 33 Chee Lan Terrace (Sands Street) had three stories with a big garden in front, which was between our house and the street. The house next to ours, about 10 feet higher on our sloping street, was rented (or owned) by a bank (Bank of Canton) which served as a dormitory for its junior employees. One of whom was a handsome young man called Siu Yu Chuan or other names, including Siao Yuk Kuen. In those days, most people didn't use standard transliteration of Chinese names like the Wade Giles system; and the Pin Yin system was only developed after the People's Republic of China was established some years later. Uncle Siu was a Shanghainese but most his adult life was spent in Guangdong and he spoke Cantonese. Even though his children all had their surname in Cantonese spelled Siu, he had a few English names spelled different ways. In any case, his Chinese pin yin name should be *Xiao Yu Quan*. But the boys all use Siu as the family name. Uncle used Y.J. Siao as his official English name in the bank, Siao being another non-standardized way of transliterating Chinese names to English. He worked for the bank as a clerk and later after the war he became the manager of the Bank of Canton in Macau. The bank's house and ours each had a rectangular courtyard stretching between the residence quarters and the back wall with a rear door. Right next to the rear wall was a modern bathroom with flush toilet and bath tub. Then the kitchen was next to a bedroom that was an extension of our main living quarters with a sizable window facing the wall that divided the two courtyards, with theirs on a higher level. The wall was about ten feet solid rock and concrete to their ground level plus another five feet or so above it which was at least a foot thick so that children couldn't easily climb and fall over it. Even adults had to tiptoe to look over the wall to see what was happening on our side.

Behind the back door was an alley; and right across that was a largely unexplored hill where I had encountered bright green-colored snakes a couple of times in its woods of mixed bamboo and shrubby plants. The bank employees could look down at our kitchen and at the bedroom with windows facing them, which occupied maybe half of the covered space between the kitchen and the main residence. I remember, for a couple of years when I was a teenager, that room was my bedroom. Obviously because of such arrangement, the young bankers and my grandma, amah, mother, and older sister, Mai, got to know one another well.

The women of my family, including Mother, Grandma, and my amah all tried to find a wife for Uncle Siu. Once, when I was maybe two or three, a younger cousin of my mother's from America (I don't know how related) came home for vacation and she stayed at our home. She was introduced to Uncle Siu and they hit it off. I think my older sister, Mai, may have played a role in their getting to know each other. Being probably three or four years old, she was the cutest one in our family. At some point before Uncle Siu met the aunt from America he had adopted Mai as goddaughter, not the Christian type, but with similar responsibilities except no religious ones. This is also not like foster children in the American sense either. But as such a godfather, Uncle Siu was traditionally bound to help Mai whenever she needed. And he later had more than done his duties by not only helping Mai but also me. At this point, an explanation of how we Cantonese (maybe other Chinese too) call relatives and family friends is in order. While we have very specific ways of calling cousins, like older or younger male cousin or female cousin, father's or mother's younger or older brother or sister, and so forth, we may refer to any family friend or relative simply as aunt or uncle according to his/her age compared to our parents or grandparents. The 'aunt' from America could be simply someone from the same village as Mother or a friend from high school or college.

In any case, Uncle Siu was not only a handsome man; he was a very stable and honorable family man. That aunt from America really broke his heart. I don't know how long she stayed in Hong Kong but before she returned to America she promised she would be back. She never came back, maybe because the war was imminently reaching Hong Kong or other reasons. Surely, before long, the war came to Hong Kong. We had to go back to my grandma's village and Uncle Siu to somewhere in China with his bank, probably not near the east coast of China, as that was too close to the war activities.

While in my grandma's village during the war, my mother occasionally went to some big city, could be Canton (Guangzhou) or Kunming (I heard that word mentioned a lot), or wherever, to meet my father. Maybe during one of those trips she introduced Aunt Pauline to Uncle Siu. Aunt Pauline was a medical student at the time. But she dropped her studies to marry Uncle Siu. After they were married they settled down in Macau and lived there from the early 1950's up until they both immigrated to the United States in the 1980's.

During those years in Macau, I started to know both of them and had spent many happy times with them in Macau. I loved them and later the boys, Raymond and Daniel, also. Both were exceptionally smart and both went to University of California in Berkeley. Raymond majored in some field of engineering, got his Master's, and for a long time worked in the engineering firm, Bechtel Corporation. He was one of the key engineers later sent by Bechtel to supervise the cleaning up of the mess after the Three Mile Island nuclear accident. Unfortunately, he died prematurely, leaving a wife and a daughter, named Harmony. Daniel also went to U.C. Berkeley, but at a younger age of 16 or 17. He majored in electrical engineering and by around 22 he had earned his Ph.D. degree. He now has his own company, married (wife named Mary) with a daughter named Frances who seems to be following in her father's footsteps; and Frances' husband is Michael.

My cousins must have gone to a catholic school run by Salesian priests because among the many times I visited Macau during my high school years, I bumped into both Fr. Smith and Fr. Ma (Machuy) from my alma mater, quite a few times. Uncle Siu, as the manager of a major bank in a small city like Macau, must have known everybody in town even if the boys didn't go to the same kind of catholic school. So we bumped into the same people. Those two priests were my favorite. Later I learned that they both became principals at some point in either St. Louis School (my alma mater) or Salesian School (where I taught chemistry during the year Fr. Ma was in charge there).

After the war and before the communists took over, my father still had some business in China. When they took over, my father couldn't withdraw his money to use it outside of China for whatever reason. That's when he sent both my sisters to China for education. Lilly got her education and became a nurse. She then married a doctor and had a son. After her husband prematurely died, she continued practicing until the immigration rules relaxed and she was allowed to go to Macau, but not to Hong Kong. Her son, Douglas was left in China for a couple of years, but later also got out. Eventually Douglas came to the States, got his engineering degree from Georgia Tech and became a communications engineer, still on his way up the corporate ladder. He is a hardworking and smart man and I'm sure he will continue to do well. Regarding Mai, she contracted tuberculosis or some illness that supposedly required Western drugs to treat. So, she was allowed to leave and went to Macau to live with Uncle and Aunt. But from what I remember of her during that period, she was quite healthy and was quite a swimmer. I think she graduated from a high school in Macau. The rest seems quite blurred.

Then, when I was in my last year of high school at Literary College in 1956, I was wondering what would come next. My father insisted that I go to college, yet he couldn't afford to pay for it. I was unsure whether or not I should get a government job to help with family finances. Then after I had passed the School Certificate Exams with honors, Uncle and Aunt agreed with my father and decided on college for me. They would pay for my college education by sending me U.S. $10 a month which in those days was quite generous. That covered all my fees with money left over for food and entertainment as well as books (mostly pirated textbooks at probably a tiny fraction of their original prices). During my five years at the University in Taiwan, the money always arrived on time. I don't remember ever having any trouble all those years. As a college student, I had no financial or family responsibilities. My only responsibility was to finish college and not to disappoint Uncle and Aunt as well as my family.

During my college years, I soaked up everything that I liked and did well in Pharmacognosy, French, and German; but I didn't do too well in other subjects, mostly C's and B's. Still I did get a BS in Pharmacy degree from the NTU with an average B grade to qualify me to apply for graduate studies in the United States. I went back to Hong Kong and taught chemistry in the Salesian School for a year. During that year, I applied to two schools – the University of Washington and the University of Michigan. The latter offered me a teaching assistantship, so, of course, I took it. Uncle and Aunt were very proud of me, so were my parents and Grandma. I saved as much as I could with my teacher's salary, most of which went to my mother, and whatever left was probably just enough for the sea fare. I am sure Uncle and Aunt helped also, and the $200 cash in my pocket for tiding me over to my first paycheck as teaching assistant was most likely from them. By then, I was around twenty-three. They treated me no differently than as if I were their oldest son, with Raymond and Daniel only preteen boys. As the boys always looked up to me, I hope I hadn't let them down.

Then, the boys grew up. Raymond was the first one to come to University of California in Berkeley to study. At the time, I was married for a year and we were living on Corbett Avenue at the Twin Peaks in San Francisco. That was in the fall of 1969 and Barbara was due to deliver our first born in San Francisco. Raymond and I waited in the hospital for hours until they sent us home. Then, the next day, Amy was born, very quietly without a peep until the nurse gave her a pinch, drawing some noise that sounded like a cry from her.

Daniel came to U.C. Berkeley a few years later, around 1972. Between the time Raymond came and Daniel's arrival in Berkeley, I was involved in various things in order to survive, including the protein from petroleum project, continuing postdoctoral research, and my getting into the importing of Chinese novelties to distribute around the Bay Area. My cousins came to visit us whenever there were holidays. Then around 1973, I was preparing to leave San Francisco across the country to New Jersey to take up a regular position as Director of Research & Development at Dr. Madis Laboratories, Inc., in Hackensack. And that was all I can remember about my cousins' Berkeley years.

Uncle and Aunt immigrated to the States in the early 1980's, I believe. For many years they lived in Irvine, California. Both Raymond and Daniel lived nearby with their families. The most important person in their lives and mine for many years was Robert Tse-Yuen Chen (nicknamed TY). Robert was the son of Uncle Siu's mentor and boss at the Bank of Canton. My father and he were friends and we simply referred to him as Taipan Chen (Big Boss Chen). Robert was the most gentle and soft-spoken big guy I have ever known. Although our families knew each other, we didn't become friends until we went to Taiwan for college. He happened to be in the same dormitory (#13) at National Taiwan University as I. His room was downstairs and mine on the third floor. He was a mechanical engineering major but his talents also lay elsewhere. He could do imitations in any language and dialect which would have us all in stitches. And he was also talented in drawing anything, besides his engineering drafts.

After Uncle and Aunt retired to Irvine, Robert's family was nearby. He was like a son to them. After graduating from NTU, he went to Malaysia to work and married Alice, a very nice and capable Malaysian Chinese woman. Around the late 1960's when racial tension became too hot, they immigrated to the U.S. First they settled near the San Francisco Bay area. Then they moved south to the Irvine area. By the time they were living in Irvine near Uncle and Aunt, they already had a grownup artistic daughter, Peilin, and smart son, Victor. By then, my family had already moved East to New Jersey to take up my second and last regular job with Dr. Madis Laboratories, got fired, and started a consultant business. Then for the next few decades I was an entrepreneur, owning my own manufacturing facility, Phyto-Technologies, Inc., for around eighteen years.

During that time, I traveled a lot and often to California. Whenever I went there, I always made time to see Uncle and Aunt, as well as to get together with Robert's and Raymond's families. Daniel, being a business owner, came to join us only occasionally with his family. It was comforting to see Robert and Alice take such good care of Uncle and Aunt. Robert was basically replacing me as their oldest 'son' and I felt completely thankful for Robert and his family, because I was far away and could not even take care of them monthly, not to mention weekly or daily. Uncle and Aunt had spent their final years well cared for and were happy. When they passed, Robert made all the funeral arrangements. I am so grateful to Robert and Alice for all they have done for Uncle and Aunt.

One thing I have regretted I don't know how to resolve which still haunts me. After Robert passed several years ago, I was unable to go to his memorial but was asked by Peilin to send a eulogy that she would read for me. I was so upset of his no longer being around that I wrote a rather emotional one. When we talked on the phone, she mentioned she didn't know my piece was so emotional and her husband Mike would read it. I felt so embarrassed that after I tried to call her a couple of times with no answer, I have not talked to her or seen her and her family since. Once again, the clueless and 'idiot boy' never left. When this book is published I'll send her a copy, hopefully she and her family will forgive me.

CHAPTER 4

Adulthood in America

HOW I GOT HERE

After receiving my BS degree in Pharmacy from the National Taiwan University (NTU), I returned home to Hong Kong and taught chemistry at the Salesian School in Shau Kee Wan for a year. This school was run by Salesian priests who also ran the St. Louis School. The Salesian School was at the east end of Hong Kong Island, less than an hour's ride by street car from my home at the west end where the St. Louis School was. At the time, Father Machuy was the principal. He was known as Father Ma in Chinese. I met him earlier at St. Louis School. He was from Mexico of Chinese descent and we had exchanged greetings in Spanish and chatted briefly a number of times. Maybe that was how I got the job right after college, even though I had flunked out twice from St. Louis School earlier.

During my teaching year (1961-1962), I applied to two universities for graduate studies in Pharmacognosy (study of natural drugs). One was the University of Washington in Seattle and the other the University of Michigan in Ann Arbor. At that time, Dr. Varro E. Tyler (Tip) was the head of Pharmacognosy at Washington but I didn't know him yet, though later, Tip and I became friends. As he was well-known in the field, he was the first one I had recommended to be the keynote speaker for the first International Conference and Exhibition of the Modernization of Chinese Medicine (ICMCM). But, unfortunately, he soon passed away, and I replaced him with Dr. Paul Coates, Director of the Office of Dietary Supplements. [see **Chapter 13: Proper Modernization...** and **LCHN**]

In any case, Michigan offered me a teaching assistantship with a generous monthly stipend enough for everything I would need and with extra to send home to my mother. So that was where I went after my one year of teaching at the Salesian School.

The year was 1962 when I left Hong Kong for America. A college friend of mine from NTU, Leo Lee, was also going to the United States to major in journalism at the University of Missouri. We agreed to meet in San Francisco and to do some sightseeing before arriving at our respective schools. We both had bought a 3-month unlimited travel-the-USA ticket (it might not be exactly called that) on Greyhound for $99. With that ticket, for the first 3 months after arriving in the States, we could travel on any Greyhound bus anywhere in the United States. So we decided to meet in San Francisco's Chinatown, during the last week of August, in the home of a family that was a friend of Leo's family. Then, we would see California and afterwards head northeast through different states until we each arrived at our school destination.

I left Hong Kong on the ocean liner President Wilson a day or two after my older sister Mai's wedding to Nelson Thayer, a Yale-in-China Scholar. The trip took about three weeks. It was my first (also my last) long ocean voyage. I don't remember much about that journey except that for a day or two on the ocean we had flying fish landing on the ship's deck. It was the first time I drank milk every day for the whole trip because we rarely drank milk at home, and it tasted good at the time. However, I didn't touch the salads, because I grew up never eating any vegetables raw. It took me another 30 years living in America before I felt comfortable eating salads, especially when they were not made at home. The passengers of the ship were mostly students like me and there was a lot of socializing and silly games in which I usually didn't participate. But I do remember admiring a music student who was going to major in piano at Purdue, I think. He used to play the piano in the lounge and did so really well. I often imagined myself playing some musical instrument but never had a chance to learn it when I was a kid, and then when I became an adult, I didn't have the patience to learn it.

I also met a German-speaking Swiss among my fellow-passengers who was going to the States and Canada sight-seeing. His name was Ernest something but I don't remember his last name. He was an interesting guy travelling all over the world staying at hostels. His English was a little choppy but he got his thoughts across. So he practiced his English on me and I practiced my broken German on him in return. And we hung out together most of the days on that voyage. However, after we landed in San Francisco we each went our own way; he went to a hostel and I went to meet Leo in Chinatown. I never saw Ernest again. We did correspond during the first year or two, but we didn't keep up. Actually, it was probably mostly me, because I always have had difficulty maintaining long-distance friendships unless with old friends like those from high school or college who don't feel slighted if we never write to one another. I have a few like those. We seldom, if ever, write or call one another, but whenever I go to Hong Kong we pick up where we have left off years earlier. Incidentally, Ernest was my first Western friend of similar age.

Leo and I met as planned, in San Francisco Chinatown during the fourth week of August of 1962, at the home of his family friends, the Chans. He had flown into San Francisco from Hong Kong via Seattle. We stayed in San Francisco for a couple of days and then we headed south on a Greyhound bus along the California Coast. I am not much of a tourist but I found the California coast very beautiful. We saw Disneyland for the first time. But I guess I was too old already and found everything rather fake. Then 16 or 17 years later when my wife and I visited Disneyland with our girls (Amy around 10 years old and Camille 4), I found it not so artificial. I guess when you see your children so excited about Disneyland, you can't help but be affected by their joy.

IGNORANCE IS BLISS!

San Diego was the last and southernmost California city Leo and I visited. While there, we decided to make a side trip across the border to see a bullfight in Tijuana, Mexico. We must have seen ads or something during our trip and decided to see a bullfight. I don't remember whether or not the Greyhound bus went to the border at that time and if not, I think we might have ridden a taxi to the Customs & Immigrations checkpoint and walked across the border to Mexico. Once on the Mexican side, taxis were everywhere. We got on one taking us to the bull fight. We each had all our money and valuable belongings in our small bag. I had 200 dollars cash that was supposed to be for my living expenses until my first paycheck from my teaching assistantship. Leo was from a better-off family and had more cash than I. Since we had no idea where we were going or knew anything about Tijuana, what if the taxi driver took us someplace and robbed us? For a while I panicked. I had watched too many American cowboy movies with *banditos* in them! But then, we got to the bullfight arena soon enough. We paid the driver and got into the arena and watched the bullfight. It was not as spectacular as I had thought. Still, the event that followed was so etched in my memory which made whatever happened after the bull fight and the little tourist stroll in downtown Tijuana become non-events.

How we got back to the border checkpoint is a blank. All I remember is we were immediately detained by U.S. Immigration/Customs. An officer took us into a room and explained we didn't have the proper documents to enter the United States, because our visas were for a single entry only. We used that up when we landed at the airport or the pier when we first arrived in the States. After maybe 30 or 45 minutes, or maybe an hour, of questioning and reviewing our papers, including university contacts such as correspondences and my teaching assistant appointment, among other papers, the officer was satisfied that we were legitimate students. He released us after giving us a stern lecture about immigration rules. He didn't even call our school contacts, as far as I know. I was 24 years old and Leo perhaps a year older, obviously both naïve and innocent. Young people at this age now can be high-level executives in government or industry. And we were just starting graduate school and traveling like greenhorns. I shudder at the thought of this episode fast forwarded to now. What could have happened?

When I was a teenager in Hong Kong, there was a widely known case of a homeless European living on the Hong Kong - Macau ferry. I don't remember the details, but he somehow got himself onto one such ferry without immigration documents. Neither the Hong Kong nor the Macau immigration let him land. For a long time he was living on that ferry as a homeless person without a country. This was the same ferry line I used to take to visit Uncle Siu and Aunt Pauline in my high-school and college days. It usually took three hours. Now the Hong Kong - Macau hydrofoil takes only one hour. I have never found out how the story with the homeless European ended. Regardless, I am grateful for the compassion of that U.S. immigration officer to let us back in.

Having been brought up in an environment encompassing some of the world's most profound religions and philosophies (Taoism, Buddhism, Confucianism, and Catholicism), I believe in fate and luck. I have been certainly lucky on more than one such occasion.

THE 'IDIOT BOY' AND THE CLUELESS NEVER LEFT

As an adult, my honest and generous nature as well as being sometimes clueless and with easy trust in others, have once in a while been taken advantage of by shrewd or downright crooked businessmen, or sometimes I shortchanged myself to my own detriment. The two occasions that have stuck in my mind involved a young entrepreneur in San Francisco in the early 1970's by the name of John Jackson (not his real name), and the other a Polish young man named Wiktor Nowak (not his real name) only about eight or nine years ago who told everyone he had a business degree from a school in Warsaw that he frequently touted as the Harvard of Poland. Wiktor was smart and charming. He was the kind who would easily see the clueless in me and exploit it when the occasion arose. Also, on some occasions, I would prematurely blurt out an answer that I later would regret, such as the one in 2011 when I was offered the Alumni Distinguished Lifetime Achievement Award by my alma mater. I initially turned it down because I was so upset after losing my trademark and was still dealing with the lies and rumors Wiktor had been spreading around and on the Internet about me. [see **Chapter 10: Alumni Distinguished...**]

John came into my life when I was between jobs/ventures in the early 1970's, after having successfully developed a process for producing single-cell (bacterial) protein from petroleum fermentation which was ready for pilot plant, with prospectus already prepared by Gulf & Western to seek potential partners (see **Chapter 5: My First Big Business Intrigue...**).

The Life of a Pharmacognosist: A Jack of All Trades

At the time of our meeting, I had just formed a consulting company in pharmaceutical consulting and translation services drawing on the wide variety of pharmaceutical, analytical, R&D, and language talents of my colleagues (especially professors and foreign postdocs and graduate students). But the income was meager, so I had to work different businesses to bring in income while my wife had to go back to work as a medical technologist. She and I had agreed to give it a 2-year try before getting back to seeking fulltime employment in my own field. One of the things I tried was being a distributor for a multilevel marketing company called Bestline, selling its cleaning products, which brought in some income. At first I went to neighborhood garages to sell them cleaners. Then, after President Nixon's visit to China, my colleagues and friends encouraged me to bring in some Chinese gift items. Since I was going around San Francisco and the Bay Area anyway, I decided to do so. That gave me more than a couple of things to sell on my rounds. I met many interesting and nice people, including small-shop owners, managers of large shops, some buyers of department stores, and a lot of hippies (in Berkeley), among others. I must have seemed out-of-place in the selling-business world, as most of the people I approached rarely treated me curtly or with impatience, even when they eventually didn't buy anything from me. Instead, most seemed to go out of their way to talk to me and rarely haggled over prices. Some even helped me with selling tips and provided leads for my future sales rounds. Now, looking back, I am sure they noticed the idiot and clueless in me and took pity on me.

I don't remember any of their names or shops but most were in Berkeley and San Francisco Chinatown, especially head-shops. However, there was one shop and its owner I remember the most, who was especially nice to me. Again, I don't remember the names. The lady owner might be 40-45 years old. I believe she was a Japanese American because the shop was on Grant Avenue and was the largest Japanese gift store in San Francisco Chinatown. From the very beginning, she treated me like I was a clansman instead of a salesman, even though she knew my name was Leung, obviously not Japanese. Whenever I made my call at her shop, which was never scheduled, she always made time for me and always bought something from me. In fact, she was one of my best customers.

My overall experience in selling around the San Francisco Bay Area was largely positive. I don't remember being cheated by anyone interesting enough to have had an imprint on my memory. Though I have never found out how the Mao buttons eventually did with John Jackson. My explanation follows. I met John in his junk yard during one of my rounds around San Francisco. He was a young hippy-looking guy, maybe in his early twenties (though I would be the worst person to be an eyewitness), definitely long-haired, skinny, outgoing, and friendly. He was obviously a smart businessman and not like the usual hippies I encountered in Berkeley in those days. He seemed to be a straight honest guy and to have a prosperous junk business selling old stuff to others to distribute to shops. Maybe he also sold directly to shops. I didn't ask, nor cared, as befitting my clueless nature. For some reason, I liked him and trusted him. He wanted to have Mao buttons for distribution and promised me he could sell tens of thousands of them. Incidentally, for those too young to know about Mao buttons, they were little metal or plastic pins with Mao's face on them in various sizes and shapes, though mostly round, that most Chinese wore on their lapel during the Cultural Revolution of the 1960's to 1970's.

Mao was the Communist leader who led the revolution that established the current People's Republic of China after driving the Republic of China under Chiang Kai-Shek to Taiwan. After Nixon's first China visit in 1972, Americans started to learn about the Mao buttons, along with acupuncture and Chinese herbs. Based on John's word, I asked my uncle and aunt in Macau and a brother-in-law in Hong Kong to scoop up thousands of Mao buttons of different varieties and sizes over a period of a few months. When the buttons arrived, he quickly sold some, maybe several hundred and got himself featured in a major San Francisco newspaper, probably the S.F. Chronicle, with a photo of himself and some Mao buttons prominently in display. We were both so excited and I immediately brought in another maybe ten thousand in probably two shipments at his request, based on his projections. All these were based on a handshake as was usually done among small entrepreneurs in those days. However, for whatever reason, he didn't make the efforts to (or simply couldn't) sell the Mao buttons. And he also never paid me for them except maybe the first couple thousand. Once, I overheard a couple of businessmen I knew (but don't remember who) casually talking about stiffing another, right in front of me, saying something like, "he deserved it because he doesn't have a clue and shouldn't be in business…" Now, when I think about it, one of those businessmen could be John. But on the other hand, that just didn't sound like him. There must be another reason John didn't pay me.

As I was the kind who was not pushy in business matters and never really enjoyed running a business, especially when there was competition that invariably would leave someone hurt. This is opposite to scientific research in which I have always demanded precision from myself and my technical staff, with no compromises. And I am known for that. There, the idiot or clueless in me would not show up, except perhaps if I was not paying enough attention. But with John, my guess is that maybe he had never dealt with a businessman like me before and would have paid me for the buttons if I had demanded, or even just asked, as any good businessman would do. But since I didn't seriously demand it and had quickly moved on, he might just have forgotten about it. Or he might have remembered to pay me but couldn't find me, because I had moved across America to take up a job of my profession in New Jersey with Dr. Madis Laboratories. That was 45 years ago and water over the dam! Since then, I have borne John no grudge or ill will.

Then, only maybe a couple of years or so ago, I found out by chance that John, after our stint with Mao buttons, moved on to other endeavors and eventually became a prominent political figure and real estate tycoon in the San Francisco Bay area. What a discovery! I called him and had a nice chat with him. We had plans to get together but I couldn't make it when I last visited the Bay Area for a dear family friend's memorial. She was Camille Chhabria, my wife's roommate in Children's Hospital in San Francisco, where she gave birth to Vince, now Federal Judge of the District of Northern California. My wife gave birth to our first daughter, Amy, now a professional cellist. Our second daughter, Camille, is named after her.

However, with Wiktor Nowak, it was a different story. He was a cunning salesman, personable, sometimes flamboyant, and very good in persuading and intimidating people to buy anything. His hero was, at that time, interestingly, Donald Trump. He was fine as long as he was selling and making money; and he would treat his people well. In that sense, he was at least better than his hero. But if for whatever reason he didn't do well, he would do anything to overcome that, including lying, cheating, and stealing. When I first met him, he already had a partner called Aron Kucharski (not his real name) who appeared to be an opposite but complementary counterpart of Wiktor. Unlike Wiktor, Aron was low-key, also likable and with a boyish charm. But looks can be deceiving. Even my wife, who is good in judging the character of people, was taken in by this pair.

They both came to the United States after having done their homework and signed a sales agreement with me to market my PhytoChi, an herbal drink based on mostly Chinese tonic herb extracts, with a minimal monthly sales of high five figures. After eight or nine months, they couldn't keep up with their sales volume as agreed and had to forfeit their exclusive distributorship which was the whole Europe, excluding the Czech Republic and Slovakia. After they defaulted, Wiktor assured me that he could catch up with the sales in a couple of months. I believed him and tried to work with him to make our collaboration successful. And I persuaded his organization to join forces with another in Europe (the Czech company that included the Slovakians) to form a more global organization because of their complementary skills and strengths. Wiktor's was fresh and dynamic while the Czech's was slow but steady and had been with us for over ten years at that time, though its sales were unremarkable.

They both seemed to agree with me. About three months after Wiktor's default, he invited me to go to Warsaw, Poland, to get together with the Czechs to sign the agreement. All these months, he verbally promised me that he would make up for his defaulted amounts as soon as we had the papers signed. When we were in his Warsaw office studying the legal documents, the original agreed-upon terms were changed overwhelmingly in his favor. Wiktor, Aron, and the Czechs were negotiating for hours trying to come to an agreement, but couldn't reach one by dinner time. So, we all went to dinner, except Aron. After dinner, we went back to the table but still failed to agree after further negotiations that night. The next day, the Czechs went home and I was totally under Wiktor's control or maybe spell. At the time, I was physically and mentally exhausted, especially after experiencing a TIA (transient ischemic attack or mini-stroke) only weeks earlier trying to get the two very contrasting and antagonistic groups (in ethics, honesty, and marketing abilities) to work together with what I thought was success until we all sat down ready to sign papers. The next day we spent all day drafting up new papers along with Wiktor's attorney. All I was focusing on during that trip was that after we signed the papers I would have some of that money Wiktor owed me to keep my company operating. My thinking was also stuck with the idea that if after I got home and found the agreement was no good I could always rescind it within three days in the U.S. But that was not correct with Polish law. Then, I protested strongly to Wiktor that he had lied to me and tricked me into signing papers to grant him my trademarks and rights to sell my products in Europe and probably worldwide. Soon after, defaming emails about me from persons (or simply made-up names) I didn't know started to arrive in the email inboxes of many of my friends and colleagues. Based on the timing and the particular friends and colleagues who told me they had received these emails, I figured out that their email addresses could only come from my Outlook files up to the date when my laptop data were stolen by someone, most likely Aron at the office, while we were away having dinner. None of similar derogatory emails later received by family, friends and colleagues had any information that occurred after that date. My whole trip to Poland for signing papers seems to have been carefully planned by Wiktor and Aron. Prior to that trip, Aron had once helped me set up a presentation from my laptop and asked me for my password.

That whole episode was a nightmare. I liked both of them and trusted them. It was painful to be betrayed by people I had trusted and liked, not to mention the actual damage done to my business also. I have learned a hard lesson. This is the worst consequence of my being clueless and an 'idiot boy.'

CONSULTANT IN NATURAL PRODUCTS

In our industry, probably others also, when you can't find a regular job or are between jobs, you hang up a shingle and call yourself consultant. I did that a couple of times between jobs. The first consultant title I gave myself was between my postdoctoral position at the UCMC in San Francisco and my first job as microbiologist at a research and engineering firm called Bohna Engineering in its petroleum fermentation project (see **Chapter 5: My First Big Business Intrigue...**) in the late 1960's and early 1970's. The second time was between my Bohna job and my job as Director of Research & Development at Dr. Madis Laboratories in Hackensack, New Jersey between 1971 and 1973. Then after I was fired from Madis less than three years later for refusing to do something illegal, I have been a consultant ever since. However, at times, I had to form a legal non-person entity in order to do business with our government. I don't know what it is now. But in those days, a real person couldn't have contracts with the government, only 'paper persons' such as corporations, companies, and the like. And AYSL is the first company I formed and used to receive purchase orders and later the database contract (SBIR Contract Phase I) from the National Cancer Institute (see **Chapter 8: David vs. Goliath: NCI SBIR Phase II Database Contract – What if ...?**). This has always been a one-man operation.

Between the 1970's and 2000's, for more than 30 years, I was known for my innovations and outspokenness. I couldn't help it because of my sometimes clueless nature as well as my approach to solving problems which is often unconventional, though creative. Even in the short time I was working for Madis in the mid 1970's, I spent only weeks to come up with a simple process for producing levodopa from velvet beans, bypassing expensive and elaborate processes using ultrafiltration or chromatography that requires big investment in machinery and complicated manipulations. Instead of trying to separate the levodopa from a liquid soup containing countless chemicals, including proteins, amino acids, carbohydrates, and other large molecules, I had them prefixed in the cracked beans so that these compounds were not being extracted along with levodopa in the extract to interfere with its further purification. And the levodopa could even start to crystalize out of the filtered water extract on concentrating the solution.

LEVODOPA EXTRACTION AS EXAMPLE OF THINKING OUTSIDE THE BOX

It was around mid-1970 when I was working for Dr. Madis Laboratories that has since changed hands a few times. The owner, Dr. Madis, had hired a new plant manager Mr. Guy Riccardi. Guy brought with him a process for making levodopa (l-DOPA) from velvet beans. For your information, levodopa was a new drug for treating Parkinson's Disease (PD) at that time. But it had some serious toxic side-effects that were allegedly caused by impurities present in the synthetic chemical which could not be removed during its purification process. According to Guy, Dr. George C. Cotzias, a pioneer in using levodopa in treating PD, had done some preliminary study with natural levodopa from velvet beans and found it to have much fewer side-effects than its synthetic counterpart; and he was interested in a source of the natural levodopa.

Guy's process made use of the reverse osmosis (RO) process to purify this product. The RO process involves the use of a membrane (like a microscopic sieve) of appropriate size through which water and small molecules like levodopa can pass but not large chemicals like protein and carbohydrates, among others. The water solution/filtrate that contains the levodopa can then be easily purified. At that time, RO machines were very expensive. So Dr. Madis asked me to look into an alternative method of isolating levodopa from the beans. I started with literature search and found a couple of patents but none of them worked. One of the better ones actually ended up making a soup and it was very complicated to separate levodopa from it. So, I designed a few experiments for my chemist to try. At the time the only chemist I had was Bob Noll. He was basically an analytical chemist, and a good one. After a few failures playing with messy 'soups' an idea came to me. Why try to separate levodopa from the protein and starch soup? Why not fix or trap the big molecules within the beans before even starting to extract the beans with water so that we would have only water and smaller chemicals without proteins or carbohydrates to deal with. So we didn't mill the beans. Instead, we simply cracked the beans into pieces or a very coarse powder and thoroughly wetted and mixed the beans with acetic acid to denature the proteins. That mixture was simply a damp mass not a mash or suspension. Then, when we poured water into the vessel with the beans and warmed them up to fix the proteins in the beans, there was no more mess. What we got was a regular extract and not a bean soup. After we filtered and concentrated the extract for crystallization, we tested the crystals of levodopa. What we found was a very pleasant surprise. The purity was already over 90%. The time we spent on this project was maybe only three weeks. Since the beans are known to be toxic only because they contain the levodopa, the chances that the purified natural levodopa containing a highly toxic chemical other than levodopa would be slim as opposed to a synthetic levodopa produced from unnatural chemicals reacting with one another to produce totally unknown and potentially highly toxic intermediate compounds that may have never existed in nature before. During my 55 plus years of working with chemicals, the conventional wisdom among chemists is that the synthetic version and the natural version of a chemical are the same as long as they are both pure. But how pure? 98.0% or 99.9%? How about the remaining 2.0% or 0.1% containing a tiny amount of some highly toxic unknown chemical? The USP/NF specifies the purity of levodopa to be containing 98.0% to 102.0%, depending on the analytical methods used. It doesn't specify 100.00% or even 99.99% (absolute purity or close to it) because the analytical techniques available are not that precise. So, a 'pure' chemical always has impurities in it. The impurities in natural chemicals are not brand new to our environment. But those present in synthetic chemicals are totally unknown to us and have absolutely no history of interacting with us. I think you should be aware of these facts.

I suggested to Dr. Madis that we patent this process. He agreed and I wrote up the process. My memory is that at that time you couldn't put just any person's name on the patent. This person had to actually have taken part in coming up with the idea or had worked on developing it, not just being the owner of a company and you are then automatically entitled to put your name on the patent application. Otherwise, the patent would be disallowed if others contested it. So, since Dr. Madis' name was not on the application, he simply shelved it. And I have never heard anything more about this project since. However, Guy knew about this process and the simple rationale behind it.

After I was later fired from Dr. Madis Labs for another matter, I heard rumors that Merck had started a levodopa production facility in Brazil to make the product from velvet beans. I was aware that Guy had been in touch with Merck. But I don't know if the reason of his contact with Merck was for levodopa production or for seeking employment. I always wonder if the rumors were true, and if so, whether Merck used Riccardi's RO process or my protein-fixing process. If it is true, I bet it is the latter – a much superior and simpler process.

I have described traditional Chinese herbal medicine more than once or twice before as rich sources of natural cosmetic ingredients in this memoir, in my Newsletter (**LCHN**) to be republished simultaneously with my memoir, in my Encyclopedia, and elsewhere. In the Encyclopedia, I actually added a whole section on Chinese cosmetic ingredients in its 2nd and 3rd editions published in 1996 and 2010 respectively. For people who never had experience or knowledge of Chinese herbs, many of them are turned off by the use of esoteric language in describing their properties. But if you know Chinese herbs and also have been trained in the sciences dealing with them, you can correlate archaic or esoteric language with modern scientific (including pharmacologic) terms. I did just that and figured out some secrets hidden in that 'mumbo jumbo.'

Hence, during my last consulting period between 1970's and 2000's, I consulted for many cosmetic and drug companies, including Avon, Estee Lauder, Roche, and L'Oreal, among others. The most memorable experience was with Avon. Its new facial treatment cream contained retinoids (related to Vitamin A). It was one of its best sellers; but it had a problem. It caused rashes and needed that fixed naturally and fast. There was no time to perform basic R&D. There were some big names in the industry at the time, including a well-known dermatologist Dr. Kligman and a Ph.D. in Pharmacognosy known around the world (see **Chapter 8: David versus Goliath: NCI SBIR Phase II Database Contract – What if...?**). So Avon started interviewing consultants. As far as I was told, it only interviewed three altogether - the above two, plus me.

In my presentation, I told them I could first give them five herbal extracts for them to test against rashes, and one of them should work. So, I was given a 3-year contract. Probably the conservative thinking of Avon's technical staff that that research would require years and not months. However, in only weeks, I gave them the five extracts. One worked. It was a magnolia flower bud extract. Avon wanted it right away. Since I was not an approved vender at the time, we had to go through one of Avon's approved vendors so that there would not be any delay in supplying them with the extract. That seemed to have solved everyone's problem. Avon was happy; so were its approved vendor and I.

CHAPTER 5

My First Big Business Intrigue: Research in Single-cell Protein Production from Petroleum

The title of this chapter means growing non-harmful bacteria that have the ability to 'eat' (or subsist on) petroleum to grow by dividing exponentially: 1 into 2, 2 into 4, 4 into 16, 16 into 256, 256 into 65536, 65536 into 4294967296, and so forth; you get the picture. These bacteria are grown in a broth containing petroleum in a sterile vessel until there are countless of these single-cell bacteria. As they contain high amounts of protein, usually 75%-85%, we call them single-cell protein. You could harvest these cells and clean them up as a source of protein. During the late 1960's, there was a petroleum glut. Oil companies, especially British Petroleum, were trying to find ways to utilize this excess petroleum. One of the potential research projects was to turn some petroleum into single-cell protein to be initially used as animal feed. But eventually it could be used as a high-protein food for humans if all potentially toxic residual remnants of petroleum were removed.

After having received my Ph.D. in Pharmacognosy from the University of Michigan, I was offered a postdoctoral research fellowship by the University of California Medical Center in San Francisco (UCMCSF) to conduct research on the biosynthesis of opium alkaloids under Dr. Einar Brochmann-Hanssen, Professor of Pharmaceutical Chemistry at the Pharmacy School. The research was basically trying to find out how codeine, morphine, and other such drugs are formed and transformed in the living opium poppy plant. We had a greenhouse on the hill above the

Medical Center under lock and key. I had a set because I was in charge of watering and feeding the opium poppy plants. So I went from research on hallucinogens as my Ph.D. thesis work in Ann Arbor to narcotics as my postdoctoral research at UCMC in San Francisco.

At Michigan, I worked on the cultivation of hallucinogenic mushroom mycelia and the isolation of potential hallucinogenic compounds from them. The hallucinogens that I isolated from the mycelium (mushroom or fungal tissue) grown in a home-made 5-gallon Carboy fermenter are close relatives of psilocybin that was first isolated from the Mexican Magic Mushroom, *Psilocybe mexicana*, in the 1950's by the famous chemist, Dr. Albert Hofmann. Using only milligram quantities of the isolated and purified compounds, I figured out the chemical structures of two of them; one has 1 and the other has 2 fewer methyl groups (1 carbon atom bound to 3 hydrogen atoms) than psilocybin. And I had the pleasure to name them baeocystin and norbaeocystin because the mushroom's scientific name is *Psilocybe baeocystis* and psilocybin had already been named after the genus *Psilocybe*, leaving me its specific epithet, *baeocystis,* on which to base the names of the new chemicals. Four or five published papers resulted from my doctoral research.

I must relate one little episode close to the end of my doctoral research which caused me a big concern. After spending many months growing fungal tissue and building up enough of the mycelium, freeze-dried, for extracting the psilocybin analogs, I almost had to start the process all over. There were at least three or four of these analogs, with baeocystin in the highest concentration, followed by norbaeocystin and then others. These compounds were isolated by separating them with column chromatography (a separation and analytical technique that separates the compounds by using an adsorbent column in a glass tube which holds on to them at different degrees of firmness when they are pushed down the column by a solvent and emerging one at a time at the bottom). It was at the final stages of my doctoral research. The solutions collected now contained only one major chemical each, which is concentrated by evaporation under vacuum from maybe 100 cc (milliliter) down to a couple of cc. At this stage, the solution would be concentrated enough for the crystal to form, especially when refrigerated. I had no problem with the baeocystin solution, because I had it in a 10 cc beaker that was not that difficult to handle. And I had at least 2 cc of it. But with norbaeocystin, I got the solution down to less than 1 cc (1 teaspoon contains 5 cc) and while I was trying to transfer it into another beaker, I knocked it down, and the whole liquid spilled on the lab bench. Fortunately, it was such a small amount it did not spill over the bench top. And as I always kept my bench clean, there was no contamination by other chemicals that I needed to clean up either. Consequently, I was able to recover most of it by soaking the liquid up with filter paper, washing (i.e., extracting) it off the filter paper with a solvent 3 or 4 times and then re-evaporating off the solvent. Eventually, I did get 2 mg of the compound and was able to determine its chemical structure with that amount. That was quite a scare. Just imagine spending months to grow enough fungal tissue to go through the extraction and isolation process all over again!

The opium alkaloids research at the UCSFMC resulted in my being co-author in five additional publications. They were based on the compounds I isolated from the poppy plant after they had been injected with chemical precursors in an attempt to trace the formation of different chemicals related to morphine. The new compounds are intermediates (including 13-oxycryptopine, 16-hydroxythebaine and salutaridine) on their way to become morphine, codeine, or other opiate chemicals. These all happen in the poppy plant, hence the process is called biosynthesis and not chemical synthesis like what would happen in test tubes or flasks.

After almost three years of postdoctoral research with Prof. Brochmann-Hanssen, I was hired by a small contract research engineering firm in San Francisco to work on a project involving growing microbes (specific bacteria) in experimental fermenters for their protein (called single-cell protein). The company (Bohna Engineering) had a contract with a promotor (Fred Lauer) who had bought a process from some Italian Ph.D. called Dr. DeBuda. Fred saw the prospect of turning crude oil into protein at that time (late 1960's and early 1970's), first as animal feed and eventually for human consumption. He believed he had the process and wanted to make big money from it, not that he was not rich already, at least outwardly.

Here is a little story about Fred: when we were maybe a year into the project under my direction, making much progress, Fred was on one of his occasional visits and parked his new Rolls Royce convertible outside our building in Oakland's industrial neighborhood, not exactly a place to park such a vehicle worth probably half a dozen decent houses in the Bay Area at that time. One of our five or six lab staff (a Chinese engineer with chemistry background) came in from the outside after lunch and announced aloud, "What happened to Fred's car?" Fred heard it, and I had never seen someone disappear that fast! But that was just Wendell's dry sense of humor.

Before I joined Bohna, its lab staff, consisting of an engineer and a chemist, had already been working on the project for months, until the project manager (named Orm Bretherick, a process engineer) realized that they were not getting anywhere. They obviously needed a microbiologist specializing in microbial fermentation. Guess what, I was just looking for a job after my postdoctoral appointment. How coincidental! That job seemed to be waiting for me. During my interview, I was appalled at the conditions under which the fermentation was being conducted. It was in the same room as Bohna's fertilizer project, grinding up rocks, with dust all over. I told Orm that I would have to discard all the results they had gotten so far and restart from scratch, including hiring new staff, starting immediately after joining the company. Orm agreed and I was hired right on the spot. Orm was in his late fifties or early sixties. He reminded me of Mr. Dithers in the Blondie cartoon, with thick glasses and knitted brow, rarely cracking a smile, but whenever he did, it was a warm smile. Orm was easy to work with and gave me free rein in the hiring and purchasing of any necessary equipment and materials for our work. He never interfered with my direction of the lab work and left it totally to me. One thing I have learned from heading a research team is that, if you are in charge and know what you are doing, without someone above you who has gotten there by warming his/her chair longer than you, to interfere with your decisions, you can get things done really fast. In our case with Orm, his knowledge of engineering and mine of microbial fermentation (nutrition, chemical analyses, biochemistry, etc.) complemented each other very well.

My very first move after being hired was having a solid partition built to separate the fertilizer project from our fermentation project. Within a couple of weeks, I hired an assistant with a fresh bachelor's degree in biology and some basic knowledge of microbiology. I did that intentionally because fresh graduates with enthusiasm have few bad, entrenched habits, and would learn fast when properly motivated and mentored. The name of my assistant was Larry Cummings who later joined Bio Rad after our project was dissolved. I trained him along with the two original lab staff who had worked on the project before I took over, in sterilization and aseptic techniques essential for proper inoculation of bacterial cultures and avoiding contamination, not that there are many bacteria that can grow on petroleum. Then, for a couple of weeks I worked with them, making sure all necessary precautions were taken to minimize microbial contamination starting from the preparation and sterilization of the culture medium (a nutrient broth), handling of the bacterial culture, inoculating it into the broth, sampling the culture during fermentation, and so on, until harvest. After those weeks, Larry, Art (the chemist), and Wendell (the engineer) were able to manage routine work on their own.

At the beginning, after hiring Larry, our lab staff consisted of three. The very first thing I did was to discard all the prior months' work that yielded useless results obviously all due to unknown, possibly contaminating microbes; and none of them showed extraordinary growth that was worth keeping for further investigation. We started anew with a few bacterial species purchased from the American Type Culture Collection - from test-tube to flasks and then to fermenters of different sizes which the process engineer (my boss and partner), Orm Bretherick, designed, based on my visualization and recommendations from the fermentation angle. Soon, in weeks, after analyzing the harvested bacteria for protein content, amino acid profile, and other nutritional chemicals, we settled on an innocuous *Micrococcus* species as our target microbe for protein production from petroleum. We then concentrated on optimizing and maximizing its ability to 'eat' petroleum to grow in a nutrient broth containing petroleum as the carbon source along with a nitrogen source and trace minerals, among others. We produced many batches of bacterial cell mass enough for basic analyses for protein content, amino acid profiles, minerals, residual hydrocarbons, and other potential toxins. All these probably took another 6-8 months during which time I hired a couple more biologists/chemists. I remember Diane, a hard worker, who had a degree in marine biology and was a college friend of Larry's. She was physically as strong as any of the guys in the lab, yet she was not a real big woman. Then, there was Bill Mulder, with a Dutch name, who took smoking breaks a lot, but otherwise was a decent worker. By then, we had moved to an industrial 1-floor building in Oakland where we had plenty of space and were ready to continue the next phase of our work. Soon, it was funding time because we were at a juncture when we needed more staff and equipment to go to the next phase. So, while waiting for funding, probably only two or three weeks, Bohna management laid off all new hires. I basically was sitting at my office in San Francisco, bored to death. When I got home every night I was dead tired. Yet I didn't do anything! I just couldn't (still can't) take boredom! I was certainly thrilled to get back to work when Gulf & Western picked up the project. And I hired everyone back and we charged ahead anew.

We continued to produce more batches of bacteria, harvesting them and analyzing them for proteins, amino acids, and residual petroleum contents, among other key components. Finally, we concentrated on working with a particular *Micrococcus* species (*Micrococcus cerficans*) which gave the highest digestible protein with the best amino acid profiles. Chicken-feeding tests were performed and found satisfactory. Samples were also sent to G&W headquarters back east for visual evaluation. The president at the time (Judelson?) even tasted it, I was told, and approved the next phase of the project. In less than 18 months of actual work (not including the lay-off and waiting months), we had developed a bench-scale process ready for pilot plant.

Then, during one of the visits of a G&W vice-president (George Urbanis) from New Jersey Zinc (a G&W subsidiary) who was in charge of our project, we talked about the prospectus on which he was working with Fred Lauer and Bohna's President, Ed Arndt. The progress of our research came up and I told him that we didn't have a process from Dr. De Buda. We basically developed it mostly during the time when G&W was providing the funds. My big mouth opened a can of worms. The G&W

vice-president wanted more information and I simply told him how I was hired and what I saw and then what I did to that point, mostly about the work my crew and I had done. He was a pleasant guy and obviously a seasoned businessman. He believed me and told me that after he returned from New York, we would discuss things in detail. I had a copy of the prospectus for a pilot plant with option for actual production at a certain output. In the pamphlet accompanying the prospectus, there were a couple of pages devoted to the transfer of personnel from Bohna to the new joint venture, AMSOURCE. It said specifically that the new company would hire a process engineer to take Orm's place and I would be transferred to AMSOURCE as chief microbiologist. When I looked at the salaries, both the project engineer and the microbiologist (meaning me) would be paid $1,400 per month. I guess in those days it would be a pretty good salary for my first industrial job. Yet, money never seems to impress me. I had been paid that amount at Bohna anyway and I never knew if that was a good salary at that time.

The rest of the contact and negotiations with George and the corporate attorney(s) he brought with him when he returned from New Jersey were fuzzy. All I can remember is at the suggestion of a friend, I engaged the services of a lawyer with a Harvard law degree. I was so naïve in business and legal matters that I let the lawyer handle everything. I probably tuned out while they were discussing boring but important stuff. Later, I found out my lawyer had demanded a 25% equity for me in the venture, and G&W simply abandoned the project. I have no idea how much he would have gotten from my 25%. However, if the lawyer had consulted me, I would have been satisfied with 1% or less.

In any case, that was my first taste of big-business intrigue.

CHAPTER 6

Herbalife – My First Experience with Multilevel Marketing (MLM)

It all started in the mid-1970s after I was fired from Dr. Madis Laboratories, Inc. that has since changed hands a couple of times, first Pure World Botanicals, Inc., and finally Naturex S.A., a French company. The reason I was fired is because I defied the owner, Dr. Madis, by refusing to follow his directions to add benzoin to podophyllin resin to 'standardize' its potency. At that time, botanical medicines (extracts) were mostly produced by traditional methods, one learned from others like in an apprenticeship. Although in the old issues of the National Formulary (NF) and the recent ones of USP/NF, there is no mention of using benzoin in the podophyllin production, the newer versions of USP/NF did specify adding benzoin in the final topical solution. It is still a major drug for treating genital and anal warts. I suspect all botanical companies used to add benzoin to their podophyllin production in those days. Nevertheless, I just couldn't be a party to that probably illegal practice, especially after I had consulted with a couple of colleagues specialized in these matters. So, I was fired abruptly one day when I returned from visiting a customer. Dr. Madis, the old man himself, did it and personally watched me pack my personal belongings. That was my second and last regular job.

After I was fired from Madis in 1977, I hung out my shingle and became a consultant in natural products, never becoming a 9 to 5 worker again, if there ever were one for entrepreneurs and independent scientists. During the next few years, I published several articles including a few on aloe vera (what it is and is not) and one on cascara sagrada, the laxative (regarding its lack of standards), mostly in the *Drug & Cosmetics Industry* magazine. Those were articles that dealt with commercial products. The first aloe vera article was written while I was still with Madis and published shortly before I was fired, and the cascara article was published a year later. They both caused a stir in the industry. Many things in the botanical industry were done for decades the wrong way and nobody ever pointed them out. When I saw them being practiced the wrong way, my one-track-mind mentality took over and I tried to start doing something about them. I didn't even think about the consequences, good or bad. Later when I had time to reflect on these, one of the reasons Dr. Madis fired me might be because of the aloe vera article. Once aloe vera gel is put into a product, there is no way for anyone to prove whether or not it is present in the product, because there are no <u>meaningful</u> analyses that can do that. As regards the cascara article, it landed me a two-year contract with the Penick Corporation, one of the three major botanical extraction companies in the 1970's, including Meer and Madis. At the time, Penick had the sole market of Casanthranol (a proprietary stimulant laxative made from aged cascara sagrada bark) but the product didn't have modern standards for cascara's laxative components while the British and European pharmacopoeias had them for years. The USP didn't have them either and yet it happened that the chemist in charge of the committee in setting such standards was a Penick employee. That didn't look good, whether by chance or by design. In any case, Penick seemed to be sincere and I worked directly with the Vice President in charge of technical matters. But the work there was not eventful; nor was it memorable.

However, two of my articles on aloe vera got some of the people selling aloe vera upset. There was nothing I could do about it, because even up to this day, there are still <u>no meaningful</u> standards for aloe vera gel. You simply have to know your supplier to be sure to buy the real one. As to the suppliers of aloe vera themselves, quite a few members make their millions selling mostly water. It's quite telling how most of the suppliers of aloe gel behaved during two consecutive frosts at the turn of 1979 to 1980 in the Rio Grande valley, Texas. Most of the aloe plants were frozen and they were no longer usable, yet the growers/suppliers reported no shortage. Only one owner of a large multilevel marketing company started looking for new aloe vera sources further south in the Caribbean, specifically, the Dominican Republic. He partnered with my friend Jaime Dajer of the DR.

I had known Jaime a few years earlier at Madis when his wife's brother-in-law, Leonard (Lenny) Esposito, was promoting Jaime's aloe vera. Lenny is a nice and personable fellow, perhaps a little talkative. Later, he and his wife Nancy and her sister Marielle (both Haitian, of French descent, with the family name of Douchatelier), and Marielle's husband, Jaime, and my family became good friends. Then, after I was out of Madis, I had quickly acquired a German client, Michael Moers. Michael was one of the pioneering businessmen doing business with Chinese companies years before China was opened up to Americans. He imported nutritional chemicals from China to the United States, and at one point was the largest Vitamin C importer from China for a number of years.

Michael was interested in supplying real aloe vera to the American market. He wanted me to develop a unique aloe vera gel product that would most closely resemble the fresh gel and could easily be verifiable. He had some prominent and rich Haitian friends who owned pharmacies and would let me use their facilities. I had an idea of making a sun-dried gel in an aseptic chamber, using nothing (i.e., no additives) but the sun's ray. However, two things made me change my mind in producing it in Haiti.

One, there was poverty everywhere, yet for lunch it was as costly as any expensive restaurant in the U.S. Our lunch expense for two or three people would probably be enough to feed a poor Haitian family of 4 for weeks. The people I worked with (top elites of the Haitian society of Middle Eastern extraction) didn't seem to even notice their fellow-Haitians' poverty and misery. They just carried on business as usual. And that was in the early 1980's. After I had been there only a few times, I noticed that there were mostly two classes. You either had it all or you had nothing. My hosts didn't seem to care. I was rather uncomfortable living with the rich who could be happy and at ease being surrounded by utter poverty.

Two, the facilities were practically non-existent. I spent most of my time with a coworker at my disposal trying to make the crudest gadgets for our experiments. I was down there maybe three or four times for several days each time, but not much was achieved. Then, during my last visit to Haiti and at Jaime's invitation, I went over to the DR after my work was finished in Haiti. We toured the DR and visited his farms, one of which was aloe vera. The difference was like night and day! Once I set foot on DR soil, I decided not to return to Haiti any more. Michael agreed with whatever I had decided.

With Jaime's resources, I was able to develop the sun-dried aloe vera gel in a couple of trips. Then we allocated a small plot next to the aloe fields for Sun-aloe production. This is the only one of two aloe vera gel products so far that is the least processed and can be verifiably tested to be real by Infrared analysis, affording a unique fingerprint. The other is our Spray-dried aloe. Any carriers or chemicals added to it are readily detected. Even up to this day, so-called standards for aloe gel are nothing but one or two chemical markers or assuming aloe vera gel's actions to reside in some combination of chemicals and minerals never proven to be equal, or even close to the traditional fresh gel. The first and last customer of our Sun-dried Aloe was a company called Nature's Way. It was the one that launched our pure Sun-Aloe in capsules without any carriers or preservatives. However, it could not compete with other aloe vera products because most were labeled as 'pure' but in fact contained only small amounts with the rest being filler such as gums, mannitol, lactose, hydrolyzed starch, and so forth. Their prices were a tiny fraction of ours. It's obvious to me they all likely knew that aloe vera gel in aloe products is not analyzable. It seems to me to be all about marketing. So, that was one of my many experiences with the aloe vera industry. I have been a vocal critic of it for 40 years. I am still one, because there are still no meaningful standards for aloe gel other than showing some irrelevant chemicals (markers) as explained above.

The only guaranteed 100% pure aloe vera is the fresh gel from a fresh aloe leaf. Unless you have isolated some chemical from the fresh gel which has been proven to have some specific activity you want to promote and sell as a drug or whatever, as far as I know, commercial aloe vera products have little or none of the fresh aloe vera's well-known anti-burn and healing properties. The overriding reason is that, unlike a chemical drug, there is no way to test how much aloe vera gel is in an herbal or cosmetic product, especially if the product is a liquid. So, most such products contain some amount of aloe vera gel, from 'fairy dust' to up to maybe 20% to 30%. But nobody can tell, even though some may claim to have 99%! Because aloe vera gel, once in the processed form (meaning removed from the leaf and rendered a liquid), is not testable, unless you design some specific bioassay for it. But even then, how are you sure the results from that specific bioassay would turn out to represent the well-known properties of fresh aloe vera gel? The only way to be sure your aloe vera product is real is to have an aloe vera plant on hand. I have been doing just that for years. We always have one or two at home. Around the mid-1980's, when I was developing the pure Sun-Aloe, along with pure Spray-dried Aloe, in the Dominican Republic with Jaime, I thought the best way for consumers to make use of aloe vera gel's well-known properties other than having a live plant nearby was to have an actual leaf around the house. This leaf, if kept in a cool dry place, would last for months. The cut at its base heals and closes. After that, it does not dry easily and the gel is inside the leaf for a long time! We might have been the first ones trying to market individual aloe vera leaves in the 1980's. I actually had written a brief description of aloe's properties and uses to accompany each leaf so that American consumers would know how to use it. But, of course, I was too far ahead of the times. That project never took off. Now, I see aloe vera leaf for sale in many supermarkets. Finally, I am glad to see it is readily available in the U.S.

My working in the DR with Jaime brought the honest owner of the MLM company and me together. Right after the first frost of the aloe fields in Texas in 1979, he went to the DR to investigate and liked Jaime's aloe vera as his new aloe source. He ended up partnering with Jaime when Jaime had only about two thousand acres or so. Eventually, he bought Jaime out when it was much bigger. Now, this company owns literally many thousands of acres of aloe field in the frost-free DR and elsewhere. Hence, his aloe vera products have been real. [see **Chapter 9: Adulteration Continues...**]

My Natural Sun-Aloe project with Michael didn't work out. However, a couple of years later, through his good friend, Richard (Dick) Marconi (manufacturer of all Herbalife products at the time), I was introduced to Mark Hughes, the founder of Herbalife. Mark and Dick both were very generous people, so was Michael, now that I think of it. At the time, Mark had FDA problems and needed a credible herbal expert to be on his team. At Dick's recommendation, I was hired as Herbalife's consultant on herbal sciences.

Dick was like a father to Mark. Mark started Herbalife because he sincerely believed in Chinese herbs. He went to Dick and asked him to produce his products for him and offered Dick shares of his company. Dick was moved by his sincerity and enthusiasm but he simply made the products for him without taking any equity in Herbalife; he told Mark to start selling the products to see if he could actually move them first. In the beginning, Mark would pick up his products and put them in the trunk of his car. He would then sell them out of his car trunk. Being honest and sincerely believing in his own products, he was able to persuade many people to buy them. So, he went back to Dick for more products, and the trips were getting more and more frequent. From my experience with MLM companies, when they take off, you have to have a big enough manufacturer to make products for you, otherwise your company would just slow down and eventually lose the momentum and fade away. Dick had a fairly big company called D&F Industries (an acronym for Dick and Fred; his partner Fred being an accountant) that made dietary supplements, like vitamins, minerals, and amino acids, for big companies; and D&F also made herbal supplement products. I suspected Mark would have his hands full when he sold his products so fast that he would have problems to financially keep his business going. But Dick was there for him, not only financially, but also kept his products flowing without interruption. The relationship between Dick and Mark was better than that of many biological fathers and sons. I have travelled with them and observed them together closely and also separately one at a time. There was never a bad word from either about the other. They both had good sense of humor and could tell jokes. Boy, could they tell jokes!

Once, I think it might be on the same Giant Buddha trip in Sichuan described below, we were in a big van (or a small bus) travelling from one site to another. There were Mark, Dick, Michael, and myself sitting in the front rows right behind the driver. We also had a film crew with us, three or four of them with all the equipment, in the back, along with a local Chinese guide who arranged our itinerary and meals, among other logistic matters. There could also be another one or two Herbalife executives with us, but I couldn't remember them. The drive was not short, nor was it excessively long. Probably two hours. All during that drive, Mark and Dick cracked jokes, one after another, as if one were trying to outdo the other. I've never heard so many jokes emanate from the memory of anyone, ever. They put us in stitches; sometimes even for some of the crew behind us, when they heard them. I admire people who can tell jokes because I myself can't remember any, hence can't repeat any. That part of the drive was memorable to me, but not the scenery nor anything else on our way between the two locations, whatever they were.

Mark was only in his twenties when I first met him around the mid-1980's and he started his business only 5 years earlier. He was a tall and handsome man, genuinely enthusiastic about Chinese herbs and his products. He had no marketers or hangers-on telling him what to say or how to act certain ways. During the six or seven years I knew him, Mark was his genuine self. During that time, his sales went from those of a small entrepreneur of tens of thousand dollars to a billion dollars! His passion for herbs and for his products obviously showed when he talked about them. Along with his honesty and boyish charm, his distributors believed him and his sales took off. That was true American entrepreneurship in my book, not the kind employing money schemes to try to extract money from the poor, unwary, or legitimate businesses. Around 1985, Herbalife's annual sales were heading beyond $300 million. Being so young and so successful, I think success had gotten to his head, feeling invincible. He got into trouble with the government, I don't remember how but it had to do with his diet products. After all, he was barely out of his teen years when he starting Herbalife out of the trunk of his car and not by cheating others or by betting on others' business failures! In any case, there were government hearings. And I understand during one such session in which he defended his diet products when questioned by an overweight politician which somehow elicited a counter question from Mark asking this politician why he was so fat. I love it! Nevertheless, the adverse publicity affected Herbalife sales that had drastically dropped below $200 million.

I was brought in as a member of his technical team because of my reputation and knowledge of herbs. Then, within months and at Dick's recommendation, Mark asked me to be on his newly formed Scientific and Medical Advisory Board. My job was quite simple: to be available to give technical support on herbs whenever the occasion arose and to go to Herbalife's rallies and talk about herbs, not necessarily supporting any particular products. I usually had my canned presentation, talking about the history of Chinese herbs, mostly tonic herbs that have dual use as food and medicine, and their benefits if done right, and potential problems if used out of context. The same thing I had been and still am advocating all these years. I was never told to promote any of their products, and I didn't. So I always spoke my mind. For doing that, I was paid very well. During my six or seven years of official association with Herbalife, I took its top executives to China a few times to visit herbal factories, institutes of Chinese materia medica, sight-seeing, and filming, among others. I remember that much of the footage of our first trip to China was not usable because, for some reason, most of us had been wearing an Herbalife cap during most of the trip, including while being filmed. So we had to take a repeat trip, though I don't remember when. In one of these trips, we were in a factory and the manager decided to let us try manning a packaging line for a few minutes, counting tablets, filling, and sealing bottles. Mark, Dick, me, and, I think, David Katzin, MD, (Head of Herbalife's Scientific and Medical Advisory Board) also, were on the line. After doing that for a minute or two, either Mark or Dick remarked that with us as workers, it must be the most expensive packaging line in the world! Mark had never been to China before. He was curious about everything and asked a lot of questions. I can't remember much of the details of our trips, as we were all over China and I had also taken other clients to China during the 1980's to1990's.

But I do remember one famous site that we visited when we were in Sichuan during one of our China trips. It is the Big (or Giant) Buddha of Leshan ('Happy Mountain'), which is the tallest stone statue in the world, though not freestanding. I wonder if there is a freestanding one. Anyway, it is over 230 ft. tall, carved out of a big rocky cliff during the 8th century, facing the confluence of two rivers in the town or city of Leshan. It was not the statistic that most impressed me; where we stayed the night near the giant Buddha's neck was imprinted in my memory. Up at that level there was a small Buddhist seminary converted into some sort of guesthouse or small hotel. I think there were maybe half a dozen in our party. I remember Mark, Dick, and Michael were among them. We occupied most of the rooms. There was nothing to do other than reading or practicing meditation if you were so inclined. Or enjoying the serenity and tranquility of the night, especially the environs, by ear, before falling asleep. So we all went to sleep shortly after it got dark. The next morning, we were ready to continue our drive to our next destination that I can't recall what. It was perhaps a couple of hundred feet between the seminary and where our van was parked. To get to our van, we had to walk on an unpaved walkway not wider than ten feet, lined by tall bamboo trees on both sides forming an arch. I still have a photo that I have taken showing the bamboo archway and two farm women (I assume) walking away from the seminary towards the door with steps leading to the parking area. There were also one woman and two men sitting on a couple of benches on both sides of the walkway. They appeared to be vendors with their baskets of some kind of food (not vegetables) next to them. The woman's bamboo pole for carrying her two baskets was resting on top of her two baskets. It was in the morning, they must be carrying them to some market.

In another trip maybe five or six years later when I was still consulting for Michael and, on his behalf, visited an antibiotic factory across the river from the Giant Buddha. After business meetings, my hosts took me to see the Big Buddha because that was the closest well-known tourist spot. I noticed the bamboo woods were all gone, so was the unpaved walkway. Instead, the path was paved. Since then, I had moved on to owning other businesses and a manufacturing facility supplying herbal supplements to other companies under their own brands. Later Michael prematurely passed, leaving behind his wife and a daughter called Anya. When I met her, she was maybe anywhere between six and ten years old, a tall and lovely girl. She was the apple of Michael's eye, and he talked about her a lot, though he was never a talker. After I started getting busier, I didn't keep up with Michael. Only years later did I find out from Dick that he had died of some sort of cancer. This is another regret (due to my clueless personality) which I have to bear the remaining years of my life, for not having connected more with Michael.

Here are a couple of episodes to show Mark's generosity and interest in Chinese herbs. When Herbalife went public, I called him and congratulated him. He told me he was going to give me 75,000 shares of Herbalife stocks. Just like that! It probably had been Dick who reminded him. Then not too long after, I got those shares. By now, it would have been worth millions. But I had to sell them for maybe less than 25 cents a share when I had a tough time during a difficult period of my business. But that helped. Well, being an entrepreneur, 'you win some and lose a lot!' as my friend and colleague (Ed Tello) used to say. He and I worked at the Franklin Institute in Philadelphia as indexers and abstractors on an International Cancer Research Databank for a couple of years in the early 1980's.

Another time was during one of our trips touring China, Mark asked me if I had something for his not being able to sleep for days. I just gave him a bottle of An Mien Pien ('Peaceful Sleep Pill') that was one of the standard common patent medicines I brought with me whenever I traveled around China with Western friends, including especially berberine pills for diarrhea when no over-the-counter or prescription drugs from America would work. A bottle of An Mien Pien usually contains 60 pills used for 5 days at 12 pills each day. I told Mark to take 12 pills before going to bed. But he took the whole bottle. He slept well that night and got up late the next day. It was fortunate that none of the herbs in the formula is toxic, as most are tonic herbs that double as food and drug, depending on usage. The key herbs are jujube kernel, polygala root, and licorice root among others. Later, when I heard about Mark's passing, the first thing came to my mind was the An Mien Pien episode. I wondered if he had taken too much of a prescription drug.

In the end, my association with Herbalife was an overall positive experience. Without Dick, Mark would not have realized his dream and built Herbalife to the point he had it when I became part of it. After I was with Mark for some years, along with several other technical experts on its Medical and Scientific Board (including my favorite, Dr. George Pigott, Professor of food engineering from the Institute of Food Science at the University of Washington), Herbalife's sales soared and eventually reached a billion dollars, then later surpassed them.

CHAPTER 7

MLM Cookies Corporation — The Company of Diet Cookies

In the early 1990's, I had been consulting in the area of drugs, cosmetics and herbs for 15 years. The companies for which I had consulted include big and small companies, such as Bristol-Myers, Roche, Moers Chemical, Avon, Estee Lauder, Yue-Sai Kan, Elizabeth Arden, Solgar, Forever Living, Herbalife, Penick, Meer, and Chart, among others. Three years after I was fired from Madis, my first book (*Encyclopedia of Common Natural Ingredients use in Food, Drugs, and Cosmetics*) was published by Wiley in 1980. It was timely because all other comparable handbooks had limited information. It has since become one of the key references for the natural products industries. Consequently, my name started to be known throughout the herbal industry.

One day in 1991, I received a call from a company called MLM Cookies Corporation (not its real name, MCC for short) in Ontario, Canada, which I had never heard of before. It wanted to consult with me in its office in Canada. Since it would pay all expenses and my consulting fee, I thought I would have nothing to lose to go up there for a day to talk to its people. When I got up there, its owner met me in his small office along with another younger man. Later I found out this man was the owner's cousin. MCC was a small direct-sales company, formed a couple of years earlier, whose product was diet cookies with sales of no more than a couple of million Canadian dollars.

My first impression was, "Here is a fat, short, and bald man trying to sell diet cookies! What can I do for him?" It turned out he had hopes to imitate a very popular product in Canada in the 1980's, called "KM" and to sell it from his own company, MCC Canada. I looked at the product and saw one of the key ingredients was potassium iodide with a whole bunch of herbs listed on its label like most such 'herbal' products at that time. I asked him what he wanted me to do with that product. He asked me if I could make a product like KM for him. I told him no, because I didn't want to make a product that would give people a high and then let them down, which would require them to take it again, creating another artificial high, ad infinitum. Besides, it would disturb their body system and make the health of its consumers worse. However, if he wanted a real health drink product, I told him I could make one for him with Chinese tonic herbs which would give people genuine tonic effects. This would later be called Herbal Health Drink (not its real name) or HH-Drink for short.

According to traditional Chinese medical practice, the *yin* and *yang* in your body system must be balanced in order to be healthy. When they are not balanced due to whatever reason (stress, side-effects of drugs, excessive work or exercise, too much drinking, smoking, and many others) you would become ill. These tonic herbs that can function as both food and medicine would supply missing nutrients in your body to restore its *yin/yang* balance, thus restoring health and maintaining it. When one is balanced one is naturally healthy and would be full of energy. There are many of these Chinese tonic herbs. They are just now beginning to be discovered. My scientific colleagues have so far missed the point in achieving optimal health because, like me fifteen years earlier, they have been viewing everything through the lens of pharmaceutical technologies instilled in us by the pharmaceutical industry. We were all trained by these same technologies in college through graduate school looking for and dealing with chemicals (i.e., drugs) and never had to deal with herbal medicines the proper way. Hence, we have always been treating the latter (herbal supplements included) as drugs, not obtaining the true results. I hope my book will help consumers to understand the point I have been trying to convey to my pharmaceutical colleagues in industry, government, and academia for three or more decades! Once they get it, especially when we start introducing true alternatives to our current toxic drugs, we will have a chance to counter the pharmaceutical industry's grip on the major part of our health care. [see **Preface** and **Introduction**]

Anyway, MCC's owner wanted such a health formula that I suggested. But he also wanted me to be the spokesman of the product. I told him I would not speak for the product unless I had control of what was going into it. He agreed and had the agreement drafted up right there in his office. We both signed it. After I returned home I would formulate the herbal drink for his final approval. Then, I would source the herbs from my trusted sources to send to his contract packer. The contractor would prepare the finished drink according to my directions specified in the production process. Before we started producing the product, he wanted to add more herbs to the drink. The final formula contained probably another dozen herbs, mostly Western herbs, for marketing purposes which I can only describe as 'fairy dust.' The final formula contained a total of 20 herbal extracts, including pure aloe vera powder from the Dominican Republic. Since we had already succeeded in developing a verifiably pure and the least-processed genuine Sun-Aloe (see **Chapter 6: Herbalife...**), we subsequently also developed and produced pure spray-dried aloe vera powder. This spray-dried aloe is a little more processed than Sun-Aloe, because it requires a step of evaporating and another of spray-drying. However, before it is put into liquid or solid finished products, its purity can be verified by Infrared fingerprinting. Most of the herbal drink products originally developed and/or supported by me contained this pure aloe vera. Now, none of them is supported by me except the PhytoChi from the Czech Republic, because that is the only product whose herbal ingredients' identity and quality I can still control, and it still has the same HPTLC fingerprint.

In this book (as well as my **LCHN**) I have repeatedly tried to make people understand herbs are not drugs. Drugs are well defined and easily analyzed. When they are listed on the label, it means you can be sure they are in the product, unless it is downright adulterated or mislabeled. With herbs, it is not so. Since all herbal ingredients are not single chemicals, there is no uniform standard to show what they are or should be. Hence, no two herbal products with the exact same labeled ingredients made by two or more manufacturers are the same, unless the two products are made by the same manufacturer using the herbal ingredients from the same supplier. Even honest manufacturers can be easily dragged into this quagmire, especially when they don't have knowledgeable technical personnel who are strong enough to resist their management's persistent insistence to cut costs. This can easily lead to accepting cheaper adulterated products. [see **Chapter 11: DSLD... & Chapter 9: Adulteration Continues...**]

In the beginning of my association with MCC, I sourced most of the herbs from trusted sources. As the Western herbs in my formula were only for marketing purposes, they all served no function in it. Only 'fairy dust' amounts were added. So, in the beginning, I could make the extracts at home and send them directly from my home base in New Jersey to MCC's contract packer. At first, we sent enough for a few thousand bottles' worth of these token ingredients, followed by enough to make tens of thousands bottles. In the meantime I had some local company that I knew make the larger extracts of the key Chinese herbs. Then one time, they fouled up and hid the truth from me. I found out, which prompted me to go to Iowa to teach a local homeopathic company to start building some simple equipment to produce the Chinese herb extracts. Even though I basically had total control of the contract facilities to make the extracts, I needed my own facilities to support MCC's fast growth as well as my other growing extract business.

In the meantime, I was able to keep track of MCC's growth by watching the amounts of extracts we sent out from our end. At first, it was around 1,000 bottles' worth of extracts per month, then 10,000, and then 20,000 per month. By the end of the 4th year of my business association with MCC, we had shipped out, during that year, 1.3 million bottles' worth of HHDrink ingredients to its contract manufacturer.

The product, HHDrink, did so well because I picked the best-known tonic herbs allowed in America at the time, and actually made their extracts closest to the traditional way. [see **Introduction** to compare with 'something' supplements] In addition, there was the equivalent of about 15% real aloe gel in the drink. At the time, many aloe drinks on the market claiming to have 98% or 99% pure aloe vera might not even have the

15% that was present in HHDrink. They can say that because there is no way to verify it, unless you believe or trust whatever chemicals they test to be aloe with its fresh gel's properties.

Since I was the spokesman for HHDrink, I went to quite a few rallies for MCC during my roughly five years of association with it. I remember having gone to those in Canada, U.S.A., the United Kingdom, Japan, and Korea. When I spoke about HHDrink and why and how it worked, I never told them it could do this or that. I simply told them to try it, based on my knowledge and experience with Chinese herbs. The distributors appreciated my honesty and frankness. They believed me and tried the product. Many liked the results they got and became enthusiastic distributors of HHDrink. And they were energized to sell it. I gained their trust and had credibility because I never lied to them. When I didn't have an answer to a question, I never made up stories to tell them why and how HHDrink worked with complicated terms or convoluted theories trying to pull the wool over their eyes. My spiel was simply something like this: Here is a healthy herbal drink made of safe Chinese tonic herbs. I know the extracts I put in it are the right ones and of good quality. But it doesn't work the same for everyone. Try it to see if it works for you.

In a short time, sales of HHDrink took off exponentially. During rallies, there were a lot of testimonials. I always had doubts about most of them, especially those from new distributors. However, there were also many who didn't give testimonials on stage, but rather, were among the usually long line of HHDrink consumers waiting to shake my hand to thank me or tell me how it had helped them. Many of them were older couples, past 60 or 70. There was no reason for them to tell me untruths. Many of their stories moved me close to tears. Many of them were probably also taking many toxic drugs and had numerous problems that were helped by my HHDrink. Often, after taking my HHDrink for one problem that might not be relieved, they found other problems obviously relieved. This is typically how tonics and other Chinese herbs work. They supply whatever our body is lacking and balance it. At lot has to do with our immune system. If it's shot, such as having taken too many toxic drugs, you are prone to get all kinds of illnesses and have entered the vicious circle of the pharmaceutical industry's drug therapy. My herbal formula (or any other properly formulated) <u>with the right herbs in their correct amounts</u> simply did what it intended to do – put our *yin* and *yang* in balance. Listening to such stories from HHDrink consumers at the time made me feel like I was following my maternal great grandfather's footsteps of helping others in relieving their sicknesses and suffering, which was my wish since childhood. [see **Chapter 1: Growing up in Asia**]

Then, in the fourth year when MCC's HHDrink sales reached around 1.3 million bottles, the owner either getting too greedy or jealous of my popularity, wanted me to cut prices. He was selling them at roughly Canadian $30 per bottle wholesale, while his cost from me was around 30 cents Canadian. I could have cut the herbal ingredients and aloe vera by one-third and reduced the price to 20 cents. He would never know, nor care, as even his technical director of sorts believed the product they were selling was just acting as a placebo anyway. One time, after observing testimonials one after another extolling the benefits of HHDrink, he told my wife he believed it was all due to its placebo effects. MCC's owner would be happy if indeed I had turned the HHDrink into an all 'fairy-dust' product, containing one-tenth of its original amounts of herbs and cut the price in half. I would make out like a bandit and MCC would still sell HHDrink at the same price while cutting its cost by, say 50% or more. But that's not me. So I refused.

He switched to another supplier that I later found out was one of the original three botanical extract companies. Most of his top distributors then left. Instead of exponential growth, their sales were stuck at the same level since, if not lower, as far as I know. After the switch, when HHDrink consumers didn't get the results that they were used to, the Company told them to take 3-4 times more. At the time I was with MCC (1992 to 1996), I had no technology to obtain fingerprints of my products yet, though I knew what I put in there.

We were in litigation for a couple of years. At the end, just as we were about to win back the money spent in legal fees plus compensations, the Canadian Government seized MCC Canada's bank account for <u>tax evasion</u>. So, it got its money first. I think we were just one or two days too late to get our money! And our legal expenses were close to a quarter of a million US dollars! Then, of course, MCC's owner changed the company name from MCC Canada to MCC Global, MCC International, or some other name, and continued their business of selling HHDrink with the exact same labeled herbal ingredients. However, physically and chemically the product was very different from mine. At the time, I didn't have my Phyto-True fingerprinting technologies yet. All I could say was the herbal ingredients I put in HHDrink were real and in correct amounts. So, I was confident and vouched for its integrity. Later, we tested the two versions of HHDrink and found out the fingerprints were very different indeed, with mine much stronger than the new version. And we couldn't verify how much aloe vera was in the new HHDrink either because there are no true tests for aloe vera in any finished product, as I have explained earlier and elsewhere in these two books. Basically, you can still make herbal products whichever way you want, and claim you have an outstanding, excellent, or pure product with 99.9% purity, etc., etc., and can legally market it. You can always fool a few innocent consumers into buying it. But they won't be fooled again. It's sad for consumers and for many companies run by people who don't understand what real herbal supplements are. They confuse them with cheap chemicals in inert carriers that can be easily produced and sold for higher prices because they are analyzable, hence their identity and quality can be 'scientifically' controlled. [see **Introduction** and **Chapter 9: Adulteration Continues... and Chapter 12: What's Wrong...**]

CHAPTER 8

David versus Goliath: National Cancer Institute (NCI) Small Business Innovation Research (SBIR)Database Phase II Contract — What if...?

It was in 1985, while I was having dinner when a former colleague from Franklin Institute of Philadelphia, Bernie Epstein called. We both had worked on a project with NCI on some international cancer database a year or two earlier. Now, he was working for Ketron, a small computer database company not far from Philadelphia. He was in charge of grant writing and routinely reviewed publications announcing requests for proposals (RFP's) from the National Institutes of Health (NIH) and other government agencies. He saw one from the NCI on building a computer database for medicinal plants with antitumor activities, basically saying the jungles were disappearing and we needed to document as many of these plants with antitumor activities as possible before they were lost forever. There was nothing about finding antitumor plants from traditional medicines such as Chinese or Indian. I told Bernie that I had no experience with jungle medicine nor did I believe it to be that worthwhile.

Then, after dinner and overnight, a thought came to me. Why go to the jungle? Doing that might be glamorous and 'sexy' compared to the dull task of investigating established traditional medicines like Chinese medicine. But in Chinese herbal medicine, there were already more than 10,000 herbal drugs documented. Among them, one could find many with antitumor activities if one knew how to interpret the Chinese medicinal records. And I specialized in recognizing potential new active chemicals for use in drugs and cosmetics from traditional Chinese herbs. So I called Bernie the next day to tell him about my idea, which was to deviate from the requirements of the original RFP. Instead of concentrating on jungle medicines, we would emphasize traditional Chinese herbs with their rich history most of which has already been well documented. While the original RFP had jungle medicines as the priority, with systematic traditional medicines only as a minor topic, our proposal stressed Chinese herbs, with traditional medicines of other countries (including jungle medicines) as a minor concern. For the non-Chinese botanical areas, I was able to persuade Dr. Richard Evans Schultes of Harvard University to be one of our three consultants, the others being Dr. James Duke of the U.S. Agricultural Research Services, also a well-known botanist and author, and Dr. Ara Der Marderosian, Professor of Pharmacognosy at the Massachusetts College of Pharmacy. Dr. Schultes is generally considered to be the father of Ethnobotany, a field based on the use of medicinal plants by native peoples.

Since I was going to be the Principal Investigator, my company (AYSL Corp.) was the intended contractor and Bernie's employer, Ketron, Inc., was the subcontractor. We submitted our proposal and out of thirteen or so companies having submitted bids, my company and a company newly founded by Dr. Norman Farnsworth along with some of his associates and assistants, won the Phase I contract, each of $50,000. Dr. Farnsworth was probably the biggest name in pharmacognosy during the past several decades. He was well connected to NCI and other government agencies. I wouldn't be surprised if he or an associate or assistant had persuaded NCI to put out that RFP so that his group could form a private company to take advantage of the database, NAPRALERT, that was well known worldwide. This database had been built by Dr. Farnsworth's group with government funds over a period of more than a decade. I believe they had expected that they would get the NCI SBIR contract. A tell-tail sign was in the wording of the RFP announcement. The qualifications of the applicant-candidate fit him and his group perfectly. Nevertheless, Dr. Farnsworth himself was not on the proposal.

While I had research and innovation experiences, my qualifications and those stated in the RFP didn't match for the most part. But the reviewers must have liked our proposal and my approach along with my Chinese herbal resources, otherwise they wouldn't have awarded us one of the two winning Phase I contracts, especially as <u>our research focus was not even what the RFP specified</u>.

The Phase I contract was a proof-of-concept endeavor and would last six months, I think. Then both companies would demonstrate their products at NCI headquarters and if acceptable, would be invited to submit a Phase II proposal. The winner of that Phase II proposal would be awarded a contract worth $1 million to build and commercialize the database. Consequently, we both submitted our proposals. Normally, the decision of which company would be the winner after submission of the proposals would take about nine months. But in our case, a year passed without any notification. Then, more months elapsed and still no word. When I called NCI, I got conflicting responses, from 'not ready' to 'both proposals were recommended for funding.' I had never heard of such a thing. I always thought that whoever won the competition would get the contract, not both. I became impatient and suspicious. Finally, I got fed up and wrote to my Congresswoman, Marge Roukema, of Bergen County, New Jersey.

After some time, I got the response that I wouldn't have gotten if I had not been so upset that I had written to my congresswoman (Marge) who also happened to be a close friend of our close friends, Drs. Raul and Alba Ludmer, and whose husband, Dr. Richard Roukema and Raul were both psychiatrists and practiced in the same building in Ridgewood, N.J. The letter from the Department of Human Health and Services was signed by Robert E. Windom, M.D., Assistant Secretary for Health, telling us that AYSL Corporation had basically won the competition, "... *Dr. Leung's proposal received a score of 770, with 1,000 being the maximum possible number of points, and was the higher ranked proposal. The program staff recommended that this proposal be considered for funding in that scientific area, an indication that the AYSL proposal is of value...."*

The knowledge we had beaten a monolithic organization was a consolation prize for me, though without the Phase II contract. I often wonder if I would have ever received any response from anyone if I had not been mad enough that I had, for the first time, utilized my personal connection with our congresswoman. I also contacted our senator, Frank Lautenberg, at the same time, but I don't remember if he even acknowledged my letter. But if he did, it would have been an unmemorable form letter from a staff member. One of my major social handicaps is that I have never learned how to use personal or business connections for my own benefits, which I have always felt gauche, coming from me. Asking Congresswoman Roukema to write that letter was one of the two or three times I have used personal connections for my own gains. Another was when I asked one of my father's prominent friends in Hong Kong, Dr. Ambrose So (see **Chapter 1: Growing up in Asia**) to help me present a proposal to the Hong Kong government for forming an international consortium to properly modernize Chinese medicines in the early 2000's. That failed due to the entrenched drug-development and drug-therapy system that for decades had a solid grip on modern (aka American) health care concentrating on modern toxic chemical drugs.

In any case, Dr. Farnsworth was bigger than life for his graduates and most people in the pharmacognosy, natural products, and medicinal chemistry fields. Almost everyone knew him. He was quite a character, often made crude jokes to see the reaction of his listeners. I respected him and he seemed to respect me because he was always courteous to me even though I was quite a few years younger. We never collaborated in our work, but were once together on the same committee for setting botanical standards which he chaired. However, that was finally dissolved without accomplishing anything like many such committees. I remember fondly at an American Society of Pharmacognosy annual meeting in Storrs, Connecticut in the mid-1970's, we were in a poker game together with Dr. Gordon Svoboda (the one who developed the anti-leukemia drugs from Vinca alkaloids at Eli Lilly) and one other colleague whose name I can't recall. Norm told a lot of jokes and we all drank, though I barely (maybe up to a half glass), as I was not a drinker. My wife has tried for forty years to get me finally to drink up to one glass of wine without beginning to talk to a houseplant. Now, I can honestly tell others that my wife is probably the only woman in America who encourages her husband to drink more. Anyway, I cleaned them out that night and was being teased about my being a beginner at the game. But honestly, it was the first time I played poker with friends for real money (meaning not play money). That night's take was probably no more than 20 or 30 dollars. Nevertheless, for quite a while I was teased as being a cardsharp.

Norm and my thesis advisor, Dr. Ara G. Paul (later Pharmacy Dean), and Dr. Varro E. Tyler, Jr. (who wrote the "Honest Herbal") were peers. He was from the Massachusetts 'school' trained under Dr. Herber Youngken, Jr. while Drs. Paul and Tyler were trained under Dr. Arthur Schwarting in Connecticut.

After I found out I had won the NCI contract bid, though without the money, at first I was very satisfied and proud of it – to have beaten the best team in its own game. But then, I felt badly about letting down a bunch of young researchers and staff under Norm's organization, because earlier at a meeting in Chicago I had met one of Norm's staff and learned that she chipped in to found Naprotech to respond to the RFP. I would have liked to collaborate with Dr. Farnsworth while he was alive. But because I didn't know how or liked to schmooze with others, I never tried with Norm. It's what I call it my social handicap. On the other hand, I wouldn't feel badly breaking up a 'scam' if the RFP indeed originated from a buddy system between government and academia that favors Norm's group. After all, Norm knew all NCI's key people. After his death a number of years ago, the natural products database NAPRALERT continues to be dominated by Norm's group and his influence – geared mainly to chemistry with no provisions for traditional medicines other than using them as raw material sources to discover and develop new chemical drugs, leaving the huge resources of systematic traditional medicines (with actual human-use experiences) untouched except exploited as source of chemicals to be turned into new chemical drugs. Their true value has never been properly tested even up to this day!

In the last few years, the topic of cronyism among academic and government institutions has at times popped up. To me, although Dr. Farnsworth's group has dominated the 'natural products' field (especially database) for over forty years, it seemed obvious there were scientists out there who thought my alternative idea was good and deserved funding, as both Phase I and Phase II reviewers liked our proposals and would have funded our Phase II research also. <u>But it was also obvious that that project was not meant for me</u>. Can you imagine if Norm's group had a higher ranked proposal than mine and his was recommended for funding and NCI didn't fund it, saying that there were not enough funds to go around? After having been in this diversified field for over fifty years and seen practically everything, including 'empire building' in academia and the 'revolving door' between government and industry, I don't think this whole episode of the NCI database contract was totally free of cronyism.

That happened thirty years ago. There were already scientists in the natural product and health fields who would have liked to see more diversity in the technologies used in these fields. The idea that there is (should be) only one type of easily identified and analyzed drugs available, which invariably would end up toxic, did not sit well with them. It seems obvious there were enough reviewers of our proposals, that liked to see changes in these fields, and saw potential in my approach, even though it was not the original theme of the RFP.

On looking back, it has been over thirty years since NCI rejected our alternative route (if not new direction) in our natural drug therapy, and 45 years since President Richard Nixon declared war on cancer. In that time, I don't see anything new that has materialized other than maintaining the *status quo* of toxic drugs begetting new diseases that require more of the same. Isn't it time to give new ideas like mine another try?

CHAPTER 9

Adulteration Continues to Be a Major Problem

One of the major reasons for the creation of our FDA at the turn of the 20th century was to fight product adulteration and unsafe food products. Around 1906, both were common.

Fast forward 100 plus years to the present, it's a similar situation, though adulteration has become much more subtle and sophisticated, with the focus switched to a rapidly growing field – herbal products or supplements and chemicals sold as supplements. This time around, the charlatans involved are much more clever and resourceful as well as much less obvious. They can be in companies of any size. Aided and enabled by the imprecise language of DSHEA, passed in 1994, it has taken them 20 years to steer herbal products towards specific phytochemicals (i.e., plant chemicals) that are easier to handle, and are embraced by chemical experts most of whom are working under the strong influence of pharmaceutical companies. Meanwhile, flagrant adulteration with pharmaceuticals still occurs, as occasionally reported in the dietary supplement industry. Because there is a lot of room to play with the language of the DSHEA, many of the herbal products can be on the market as long as they don't claim that they can cure cancer, diabetes, obesity, or the like. And, if these products don't cause serious harm that attracts the attention of the FDA, their purveyors can continue to sell them and make lots of money, despite the fact that these products may have little or no herbal elements in them. Some of them may get caught when they become too brazen selling adulterated or mislabeled product. But the penalties are seldom harsh enough to deter their continuing the operation, and they may then simply switch from one type of product to another to continue.

Also, a common practice has been to make sure the products are safe by adding only token amounts of herbs, with the rest of the products consisting of inert fillers and other excipients (carriers, diluents such as hydrolyzed starch, sugar, gums, and preservatives); or to put a predetermined (standardized) amount of specific phytochemicals in the products, whether or not these chemicals contribute to the herbs' traditional effects, the rest again being carriers. This way, the consumers don't get hurt and the regulators seldom do anything about it. That's before there were any serious attempts to guarantee the identity and quality of herbal products by the industry or the regulatory agencies. For a long time, the prevailing wisdom has been 'standardization' of herbs and herbal products. This means that you pick a chemical in an herb that's either in predominant amount or has been identified and tested to have certain biological effect such as anti-inflammatory or analgesic, yet may have nothing to do with the normal- and safe-use properties of the herb. But as long as extracts of the herb contain a measurable amount of this chemical, it is considered the gold standard for that herb. As there have been no alternatives to this rationale for the past 20 plus years, any specific chemical(s) identified in an herb may quickly become the 'standard' identity and quality marker for that herb, including ginseng, turmeric, tea, coffee, 'ginkgo biloba' and St. John's wort, among others.

This has encouraged extract manufacturers, especially those in China and India, to produce 'extracts' with extremely high amounts of standardized chemicals. Some of these chemicals, often labeled as "plant extracts" are frequently sold in their pure chemical forms. For example, luteolin in 98% purity from peanut hull is basically a pure chemical, so is resveratrol (98% pure) from Japanese knotweed (aka the Chinese herb *hu zhang* from *Polygonum cuspidatum* root & rhizome). When a standardized amount of any of these chemicals is used in an herbal supplement product in a base of carriers or fillers (but without any herbs), the product is sometimes marketed and sold as an 'herbal' supplement. Since these chemicals are present widely in plants (foods & herbs), the herbal supplements containing them can be labeled any way the marketer/manufacturer desires, especially when the company can add some token but analyzable amounts of the herb powder or extract to meet some claimed herbal content besides the pure chemical added. [See **Introduction** for example of such products discovered by New York Attorney General]

When my major customer switched to a new supplier for both the products my company had been supplying it, I thought the supplier(s) would be technical and sophisticated enough to at least come up with some decent imitations. If not 75%, may be 50% or even 25%? But to my surprise, that was not the case. After losing my business, I was so shocked and disappointed that I didn't think of comparing our original products with the new ones from our customer's new supplier for maybe a year. My thinking was, why bother, as I had already lost my business. However, eventually I changed my mind and I was curious to actually see for myself what those imitations looked like. So, I obtained samples of both products being sold in Europe and in the U.S. and had them analyzed along with the original products made by my own company. The analyses were performed at Charles University in the Czech Republic, Europe, and separately in the U.S. by an independent laboratory. Indeed, the results showed the imitation products were obviously not the same as our original products that had been on the market for over twelve years before being replaced by the new imitation/adulterated products. Since then, the new imitation products have been on the market for close to ten years. Consumers have been buying them all this time without having any inkling what they actually contain, despite the herbal ingredients on their labels remaining exactly the same. The thing that shocked me the most was how one of the products looked. This product is made up of only two ingredients – goji (lycium berry) extract and licorice flavonoid extract. My customer's new supplier must have been making out like a bandit. The photograph here consists of four sets of fingerprints in four different conditions each showing different types of chemical components present in it based on their polarities. For simplicity, polar chemicals have strong affinity for water and vinegar. For example, water-soluble chemicals such as sugar, citric acid, and ascorbic acid (Vitamin C) are polar while oil-soluble chemicals such as oleic acid, sterols, and vitamin E are nonpolar.

Our comprehensive fingerprints of the genuine (PT) and the imitation/adulterated (non-PT) products show such a contrast that one doesn't need to be a trained expert to tell the difference.

Furthermore, some herbal products do contain harmful herbs or concentrated chemicals from herbs which are basically used out-of-context, especially if they are derived from treatment herbs that have no history of being safely used as supplements (tonics, foods, and/or teas). Since such modern usage has no long safe-use history, these new products are not much better than modern drugs. Their safety or toxicity is not known for decades to come as opposed to most traditional herbs such as TCHM whose safety or toxicity has been established over centuries or millennia of human clinical experience. However, in this case, toxicity is not the issue because whatever herbal elements are present in the imitation (non-PT) product, are not much more than 'fairly dust' compared to what's in my product (PT). It won't harm you. But will it benefit you?

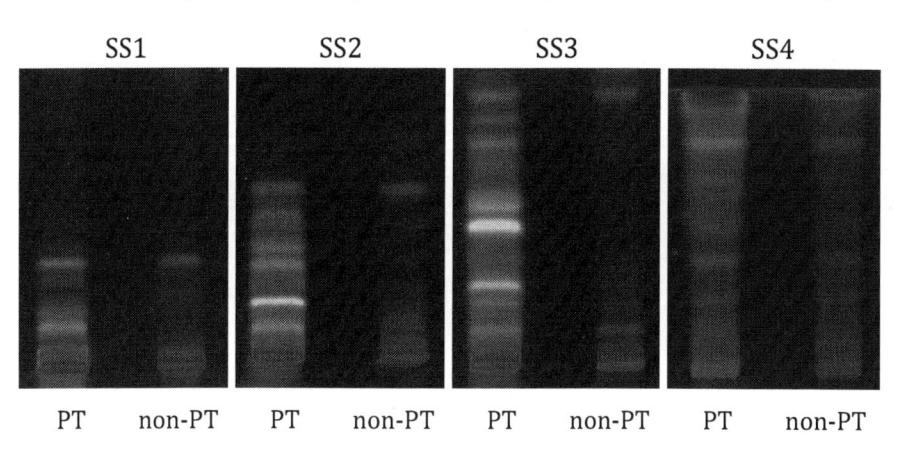

SS1	SS2	SS3	SS4
PT non-PT	PT non-PT	PT non-PT	PT non-PT

The 4 photos are fingerprints of analyses using a technique called thin-layer chromatography (TLC). The 4 solvents systems (aka mobile phases), namely, SS1 to SS4 represent 4 different conditions. Together, they separate most of the important chemical components present in herbs and foods. Each of the bands on the lane represents 1 or more chemicals. The two samples being analyzed and compared are our product (PT) and an imitation product supplied to our client by its new supplier which is labeled "non-PT" for comparison.

It is quite obvious that the adulterated or imitation product is standardized to a marker chemical (some sort of flavonoid) appearing as the highest band in 3 of the 4 solvent systems and in a concentration not even as strong as the same flavonoid (one of many other compounds) which is also present in our product. You may ask, "How can 2 products with the exact same formula be so different? The reason is that there are no unified universally agreed-upon identity and quality standards for herbs and herbal products! And the underlying real reason is that for many decades we have been applying inappropriate or downright wrong technologies developed specifically for chemical drugs to complex natural materials that include herbs and foods! Both are the same type of natural materials. One is edible while the other sometimes edible. However, if you don't know that a particular food is toxic from prior education or experience, eating it may kill you; same with herbs. And we don't need to analyze its chemicals to determine its edibility. Just imagine trying to identity a food like orange or apple using the pharmaceutical industry's chemical technologies. Should we pick malic acid for apple and citric acid for orange, or another chemical among the countless others also present in either fruit? I have often been talking and writing about this problem for decades and you can read about this in my republished **LCHN**. However, so far most of my technical peers don't seem to pay heed for obvious and sometimes not so obvious reasons as described in the **Preface** to my **LCHN** and elsewhere here and in my Memoir. The not-so-obvious reason is, as scientists specializing in some field involving chemistry, we have been taught to use the drug industry's chemical approach for natural products, from college through practical experience on the job, whether or not they are pure chemicals or complex multi-chemical herbs; and we seldom think of doing otherwise. I myself didn't come to believe that we had been trying to fit a square peg snugly into a round hole for over 40 years until 15 or so years ago. Then all of a sudden, my thinking changed which eventually led me to abandon the pharmaceutical way for treating complex herbs. Hence I understand why my colleagues are still doing the same thing that is leading us deeper and deeper into a vicious circle. The other reason, sadly, is that I believe many of my scientist-colleagues are not free to speak up due to their connections to the pharmaceutical industry and its interdependent network of associates that are holding our health care hostage. Otherwise how can any intelligent human being consider it logical to arbitrarily pick a chemical in an herb and honestly believe that this is the same as the herb that has been known and used for centuries for some indications or benefits? We don't do this with complex foods, to which many Chinese tonic herbs belong. The end result of this use of the wrong technologies on complex herbal materials and treating them as if they were pure-chemical drugs, encourages adulteration and expediency in the production and marketing of true herbal supplements.

CHAPTER 10

Alumni Distinguished Lifetime Achievement Award from the College of Pharmacy, the University of Michigan — Who would turn it down?

This 'Idiot Boy' did (see **Chapter 1: Growing up in Asia**)... at least initially.

It was in March, 2011 when I received a phone call from my thesis advisor, Dr. Ara G. Paul, Dean Emeritus of the College of Pharmacy at Michigan. He asked me if I could send him my up-to-date curriculum vitae. I said I would and forwarded it via email along with copies of two of my most recent papers. One was on the historical toxicity documentation of Chinese materia medica, highlighting its toxicity and safety, which was an invited review for the journal, Toxicologic Pathology. The other was for the Journal of AOAC International, introducing our patent-pending Phyto-True technology for the correct handling of complex botanical materials, especially traditional medicines like Chinese herbs, as opposed to the relatively easy identification and quality control of pure chemical drugs. A year or two earlier, I had also forwarded to Ara a complete set of my Newsletter, *Leung's (Chinese) Herb News* (published between 1996 & 2004, total 42 issues), after I had prepared a few sets for some of my special colleagues so that they would have it handy when researching herbal medicines or supplements. This newsletter (**LCHN**) is now simultaneously republished with my memoir, renamed ***Are Drugs Better Than Herbs?*** *An Insider's Scientific Look at Drugs and Herbal Supplements*. This Newsletter has addressed practically all issues relating to botanical or herb research, identity, quality, safety, toxicity, commercial practices, adulteration, poor research, and many others. However, throughout my writings I have been critical of the pharmaceutical industry. It is my strong belief and opinion that they have been overcharging consumers, concentrating only on one aspect of science (i.e., chemistry), ignoring or suppressing traditional herbal medicines, using them only as raw materials for isolating chemicals and developing them into more chemical drugs along with their inherent toxic side-effects. These side-effects require more drugs to counter, in a continuing vicious cycle, though less so as synthetic drugs that are brand new to our planet.

Ara and I talk on occasion, but we seldom, if ever, engage in small talk. Having been raised in the traditional old-fashioned Confucian way of respecting teachers and elders, it took me many years before I finally started addressing him by his first name. I owed Ara a lot, not just for offering me a teaching assistantship, sight unseen, without which I would not have been able to afford to go to Michigan to pursue my graduate studies. What I most admire about him is his mentoring style. He never micro managed me but allowed me plenty of freedom to do my own thing and to make mistakes. Yet, whenever I needed his advice he was always ready to help. I feel so fortunate to have had my doctoral training at Michigan under Ara, especially as I arrived at a time when the Department of Pharmacognosy was new and superbly equipped. That gave me the opportunity to acquire a broad scope of first-class training with the most advanced scientific skills. Later, after I was on my own and had my own research projects and laboratories, I was able to successfully mentor younger scientists and interact with others trained in other academic institutions. I was also able to recognize and distinguish excellence from mediocrity in their expressed thoughts and work. I have also learned from working with, or mentoring, scientists both with and without advanced degrees (PhD or MD) and found out that some with advanced degrees are not necessarily better than those without; they are often not smarter or more skilled than ones without them either, especially when they tend to assume an air of superiority even when working in a field outside of their expertise such as traditional herbs.

Around the time of Ara's phone call in 2011, my business was not going well. We had lost two major products due to my major client's switch to less expensive ones (see **Chapter 9: Adulteration Continues...**); and I was trying to deal with a new client who had defaulted in our original contract and had tricked me into signing new papers giving him rights to sell my PhytoChi under the Earth Power label worldwide and we were actively engaged in litigation. So when Ara called that March, I was too preoccupied to ask him why he wanted my CV; and he didn't volunteer the information. Then, two weeks later, I received a call from the Dean of the school at that time, Dr. Frank Ascione. He told me the school wanted to honor me with an Alumni Distinguished Lifetime Achievement Award for 2011 and asked me if I would accept it. Being totally preoccupied with having lost my major client that represented 80% of my business and actively involved in litigation over trademarks and distribution rights with my new client, I told Dean Ascione that I could not see myself accepting such an honor after making a mess of my business. He told me that the School was honoring my technical accomplishments and not my 'business acumen' (his exact words) and told me to think about it over the weekend and get back to him. He also offered to postpone the award a year and make it for the year 2012, should I not accept it for 2011.

The conversation was on Friday morning. After I told my wife and daughters later that day, they thought I was crazy not to accept such an honor outright. So, on Monday morning, I sent an acceptance email to Dean Ascione, reproduced below:

On 3/21/2011 10:28 AM, Albert Y. Leung wrote:

Hi Frank,

Thanks for offering me the Distinguished Alumnus Award. It's such an honor!

After talking with my family over the weekend, I have decided not to keep you waiting any longer for my response.

I will accept the award with humility, for my family and for the continued scientific advancement of herbal medicine.

I have always been proud of being a UM graduate. Now, I feel like a son who has done something extraordinary that makes his parents proud.

As a UM graduate, I want to continue to make my alma mater proud of me.

Please advice what I have to do for accepting the award on June 4 in Ann Arbor.

Best regards,

Al

Due to my mental handicap, this was not the first time I was on a one-track mind and made regrettable decisions. There have been many others, though not as memorable, of which my family or friends reminded me at the right time and brought me back to reality. Other times have resulted in losing business and friends. Now looking back, I think my father's calling me 'Idiot Boy' might have some rationale in it. [see **Chapter 1: Growing up in Asia**]

CHAPTER 11

Dietary Supplement Label Database (DSLD) — Not for Herbal Supplements

The main purpose of this database is to provide consumers with information on the ingredients listed on product labels so that they can pick products with knowledge and confidence from an increasingly confused supplement market. That is an excellent idea, but <u>only</u> if all dietary supplements were based on chemicals or are simply isolated chemicals already officially approved, such as specific amino acids, vitamins, and minerals, among other nutritional chemicals. But there is a major problem! The Dietary Supplement Health and Education Act (DSHEA) of 1994 does not clearly define what exactly constitutes an herbal supplement.

Is an herbal supplement an herb or a plant, a leaf or a root? Or is it a chemical from an herb or plant? Right now, the answer can be both yes and no. Consequently, this DSLD is not useful for consumers when trying to deal with the most controversial and confusing class of dietary supplements – the herbal supplements. With no precise definition of what an herbal ingredient is, how can consumers select herbal supplements based on their labels? Thus, take 'ginseng' for example. It is now a household word in America. Yet few Americans of non-Chinese (or even Chinese) origin bother to find out that there is more than just 'ginseng.' Ginseng has more than one type. The two most common are Asian ginseng (*Panax ginseng* root) and American ginseng (*Panax quinquefolius* root), but with different properties. The former has been used for over two thousand years in China while the latter was only introduced to China in the 18th century by the Jesuits from Quebec, Canada, believing it was the same ginseng used in China. It took the Chinese only

3-4 decades to find out, through actual use, that it was not the same as the ginseng found in China (aka Asian). This had different properties and was later determined to be from another plant that we now know as American ginseng. The two types of ginseng (root) have some basic different clinical properties: American ginseng is cooling and has *yin* properties (e.g., static & passive) similar to Asian ginseng leaf, while Asian ginseng root is warming and has *yang* properties (e.g., active and dynamic). Which one, then, is the ginseng supplement? Is it a chemical from one of the two major ginsengs like ginsenoside R_{g-1} (reportedly CNS stimulant) among dozens of ginsenosides, or is it all its ginsenosides including ginsenoside R_{b-1} (reportedly CNS tranquilizing) the ginseng supplement? Or is it its polysaccharides known for their beneficial effects to the immune system the ginseng supplement? It can be a true herbal supplement made with a traditional extract of American ginseng or Asian ginseng, be it a tincture or a hot-water extract, which contains all the above chemical components.

No matter how you look at it, there is no way to tell from the product label what a "Ginseng Extract" or "*Panax ginseng*" or "*Panax quinquefolius*" actually is, unless there are uniform, <u>universally agreed-upon standards</u> for each type of ginseng ingredients. Most of the herbal supplements selling the chemicals from herbs are not really traditional herbal products (herbal supplements); they are more appropriately called chemical supplements or drugs that may or may not be protected by the DSHEA. During the last five to ten years, traditional Chinese herbs have been rapidly trending towards chemicals. Ginseng extracts have become 98% ginsenosides that are basically a mixture of pure chemicals. Cured fo-ti extracts now contain high concentrations of tetrahydroxystilbene glucoside (THSG), a compound closely related to resveratrol; and extracts of *huzhang* (*Polygonum cuspidatum* root) with 98% of resveratrol are now becoming common. What I am afraid of is that the true traditional practice of Chinese herbal medicine will soon be abandoned and another 'scientific' enterprise imitating the pharmaceutical industry with its interdependent associates would take its place, promoting and selling chemicals disguised as 'herbal' supplements, unless we are aware of this and stop buying them now.

All this is due to scientists' failure to recognize the fact that herbal supplements are foods and should be treated as such; they should not be treated as drugs for expediency, generating irrelevant 'scientific' results. How scientific can these results be when you use a mixture of mostly <u>unknown</u> chemicals (instead of a pure chemical, like a drug), and expect to get good results? We were all initially set up to fail. We legally defined herbal supplements as foods and yet right from the start we handled them and started to define them using drug technology. There were no appropriate technologies to deal with herbs and/or foods when DSHEA was passed in 1994. The following is how it defines "dietary supplement" as containing dietary ingredients, some of which I have underlined below. These ingredients are obviously derived from natural sources, but different from the already approved vitamins, minerals, amino acids, and metabolites. It does not distinguish whether these ingredients are equivalent to one single chemical entity, two, or more than two:

> *DSHEA defines the term "dietary supplement" to mean a product (other than tobacco) intended to supplement the diet that bears or contains one or more of the following dietary ingredients: a vitamin, a mineral, <u>an herb or other botanical</u>, an amino acid, a <u>dietary substance</u> for use by man to supplement the diet by increasing the total dietary intake, or a <u>concentrate</u>, metabolite, <u>constituent</u>, <u>extract</u>, or <u>combination of any of the aforementioned ingredients</u>. Furthermore, a dietary supplement must be labeled as a dietary supplement and be intended for ingestion and must not be represented for use as conventional food or as a sole item of a meal or of the diet. In addition, a dietary supplement cannot be approved or authorized for investigation as a new drug, antibiotic, or <u>biologic</u>, unless it was marketed as a food or a dietary supplement before such approval or authorization. Under DSHEA, <u>dietary supplements are deemed to be food</u>, except for purposes of the drug definition.*

This is the most ambiguous definition of an herbal or botanical material that I have ever seen! Yet it is law! I guess it must have been written by lawyers based on faux science or 'flexible science' that is open to legal interpretation. As I have been pointing out for the past 20-30 years up to the present, we still have no idea what an herb, botanical, dietary substance, a concentrate, a constituent, or an extract is, <u>unless</u> we arbitrarily treat these complex materials as distinct, pure chemicals by picking some chemicals we like in them and call them herbs. Indeed, we have been doing exactly that for decades and continue to do so. The DSHEA, in one single sentence (the last above), treats dietary supplements as food, but at the same time it handles them as drugs. It is this ambiguity that generates so much confusion and controversy in the field of dietary supplements – legally they are considered food but at least practically they are treated as drugs. You can't simply treat a food (any food) as a drug, because there is no scientific way to define and analyze it using drug technology, and expect the results to be relevant for the food. No wonder 'ginseng' has been researched endless times, generating countless publications during the past decades, yet we still can't tell what 'ginseng' is. Because we have been treating 'ginseng' as drugs and/or chemicals! You can't simply test orange for its citric acid and call that chemical an orange or analyze apple for its pectin content and call pectin an apple. But that's pretty much what we have been doing with herbs and herbal supplements for decades and have been calling it science. I have written and spoken about this many times for over 25 years (see **LCHN**). Repeating it here makes me feel like a broken record.

Whoever drafted the DSHEA succeeded in making the subject so confusing and complicated that it has fooled even the vast majority of scientists. It should not be easy to confuse so many experts (legal & scientific) for so many years. But it has been. Many scientists consider drug therapy scientific and herbal therapy nonscientific. Little do they realize their modern drug therapy is not, in my view, scientific at all. [see **Chapter 12: What's Wrong...**] The true herbal supplements have better safety and efficacy records than modern drugs that give us increasingly more and more new diseases because they all have side-effects, mostly the toxic kind. Once in a blue moon, some of the side-effects produce something useful and totally unexpected, despite the fact that the original efforts to produce the drug were 'scientifically' well-planned and well-executed using the pharmaceutical industry's drug development and therapy process. Viagra (Sildenafil) was discovered this way while trying to develop a new drug to treat hypertension and angina pectoris which had the side-effect of causing penile erections but not much benefit for the original diseases. So, the manufacturer decided to use "drug repositioning" to use sildenafil to treat erectile dysfunction and marketed it under the name of Viagra. But Viagra is simply another modern toxic drug popped up by chance, while scientifically being developed for something else. There goes your scientific claim for modern drug development! It has been out in the market for only about two decades, and no one knows what serious human consequences it will bring given another decade or two. What kind of science is that? Yet, prior to its discovery, the medical and pharmaceutical establishments dismissed the idea that any drug like Viagra that caused erection in men could ever exist. They probably still say that until they find a way to patent some of the male formulas from traditional herbs.

When the government asked for comments in order to justify spending more money and efforts to build this DSLD, it sent out requests for comments to industry and elsewhere like academia and I assume selected consumers as well. I received the email notice in my Inbox. After I read it, I couldn't believe what the Office of Dietary Supplements and National Library of Medicine were trying to do by building this DSLD. From my personal experience, ingredient labels are only appropriate for chemical supplements such as vitamins and amino acids, but are useless for herbal supplements. The reason is that the former are clearly identified and defined chemical entities like drugs and there is no ambiguity as to what they are. On the other hand, the latter (herbal supplements) are mostly complex natural materials that contain many chemicals. Just using a name (extract, herb, substance, or botanical to refer to ginseng and other herbs or their extracts) does not define any of the complex multi-chemical dietary ingredients. Thus, a supplement label containing ascorbic acid and tryptophan has no ambiguity. But one containing turmeric extract and astragalus extract is meaningless for the DSLD, hence for consumers, because two products with the exact same label can be drastically different if produced by two different companies. I have written about this in **LCHN #22 (Sept/Oct 1999)** and in **LCHN #19 (March/April 1999)** simultaneously republished with my **Memoir** in a single volume. That was 19 years ago, but its information is still true and relevant! To get an idea of what two products with the exact same herbal ingredients on their labels look like, see their fingerprints in **Chapter 9: Adulteration Continues to be a Major Problem.**

I think ODS and NLM are wasting their time, efforts, and tax-payers' money in continuing to compile this DSLD unless they exclude herbal supplements from it. The herbal supplements part can be deferred to a later date after the confusion of herbal ingredients is resolved. Since there are no specific identity standards for herbs or botanicals, any botanical name, even with a specific plant part as well as some extract (solid, powdered or tincture) on a label is not enough to pinpoint what that particular ingredient is. Thus, two such herbal supplements with the exact same herbal ingredients on their label may be totally different. So I was very concerned. I lost my business because my major client, a billion-dollar-plus company, switched suppliers. It switched from my products to those of another supplier that sold them the same products with the exact same ingredients on the label, but which turned out to be very different from mine indeed. So, I sent my questions and comments directly to the key expert in charge of standards at the ODS, asking him to forward my email to the right party handling the DSLD comments. He did, but to some contractor working for ODS, in charge of entering data, I assume, but with no technical feedback. I did receive an acknowledgement of receipt of my letter from this contractor, but absolutely nothing else. That was more than a year ago! What happened?

This was not the first time I commented on the imprecision with which herbs and related complex natural materials have been treated over the past several decades. We are still doing the same. This has prompted me to appeal to the general public to work with me to weed out bogus herbal supplements by analyzing their fingerprints and comparing them with those of genuine products.

CHAPTER 12

What's Wrong with Drugs and Herbal Supplements?

In this chapter, I am going to describe a disruptive concept that I have held for at least fifteen years but never before published in its entirety. To help you understand it, I want to explain a couple of things that are essential for you to know.

Modern drugs are chemicals. They are well identified and defined. Thus, aspirin is aspirin and not another painkiller like Tylenol or morphine. Herbal supplements are naturally derived medicines or foods. They are all complex natural materials. They contain not just one or two chemicals, but many, actually countless. Among the countless chemicals present in them, the majority are unknown and unidentified. Therefore, no one single chemical in these natural foods and herbs (or one isolated from them) can claim to hold their properties and attributes as known and documented through millennia which is how we know the foods we eat and the herbs we ingest. Although we identify and assess aspirin by chemical analyses, we can't identify food and herbs by their contained chemicals such as analyzing pectin or ascorbic acid in apple and call either chemical 'apple,' nor can we analyze ginseng's ginsenosides among many other chemicals also present (e.g., polysaccharides, sterols, pectin, biotin, choline, oleanolic acid, etc.) and call any one particular chemical or group of chemicals 'ginseng.' Yet we have been doing just that for the past many decades. This wrong approach – using technologies developed specifically for chemicals and drugs on complex foods and herbs has so far produced inconsistent or irreproducible results that have been generating much controversy.

You probably have never thought there is anything wrong with drugs. Herbal supplements, maybe, as that is the general line of thinking among scientists and the general public. I used to think the same, until about fifteen years ago. Yet during most of my life, I have been intimately involved in herbs and drugs, being born into an environment of Chinese herbal medicine and then educated in modern pharmacy and pharmacognosy as an adult. For over fifty years of my adult life, I have been practicing my profession involving natural products, mostly as an independent thinker and researcher, happily pursuing my scientific career as other scientists, contributing my share of published achievements in my profession. Then, around 2005, I started to realize both drugs and herbs have a lot in common but also some distinctly unresolvable differences. [see **Preface** and **Chapter 1: Growing up in Asia**]

There are things in this chapter some of my drug colleagues and the general public may not like to hear, because they believe drug therapy is advanced science but herbal medicine is still stuck in the dark ages. However, after I have explained the whole topic and when the dust settles, I think you'll agree with me.

The continuing processes of drug development and drug therapy need to be slowed down, and we have to reset our thinking. We can't continue to let a tiny minority exploit the rest in the name of free enterprise. This drug therapy part of our health care is a clear example. In a period of seven or eight decades, it has become a self-generating money-making machine at the expense of consumers, no matter what drugs it produces and the miseries they cause. The rest of our society seems to offer no resistance.

I believe it is due to the brain-washing by the pharmaceutical industry of our younger generations starting at a tender and vulnerable age. It all began in the 1980's after drug advertising was allowed into our homes through television, followed by the increasingly easy access to drugs supplied by the industry. Over the decades, pain-killers got stronger and stronger because of synthetic modifications of natural ones along with brand-new manmade ones. Thus, morphine, the first natural painkiller isolated from the opium poppy, was modified to become heroin (diacetylmorphine) that is three to five times stronger than morphine. For years, heroin has struck fear with the general population because its addiction has killed many people. Then, Fentanyl was synthesized. It is 50-100 times stronger than morphine! And there are many such chemicals with even stronger action than Fentanyl already synthesized. In fact, the problem has gotten much worse. Addiction to Fentanyl, Oxycodone, and other readily available, over-prescribed drugs has become an epidemic in the U.S. Do we need all these strong medicines? Incidentally, another chemical called W-18 has also become increasingly reported online; it is allegedly 100 times stronger than Fentanyl, not just morphine, but Fentanyl itself! Thus, this W-18 is basically 5,000 to 10,000 times stronger than morphine! In order to fight this epidemic, we need to look deeper into our collective psyche, our roots, and what family values mean. It's not just more treatment and enforcement, or the usual rehabilitation. Many of these efforts are not actual long-term solutions. We need to look at the source of these chemicals and the incentives to develop and produce them. As long as these drugs are available, legally or illegally, with profit incentives for people (e.g., chemists, drug companies & marketers) to exploit the sad plight of the victims, this epidemic will not go away. Only in terminally ill patients with intense pain should these strong painkillers be used.

In addition to the above well-publicized epidemic, there is another one creeping up on us for decades. It's our older people's using way too many drugs. Statistics are difficult to pinpoint, but I think it is safe to say that 40% to 50% of seniors now take more than half-a-dozen prescription drugs daily to barely function, or to just stay alive. And prescribing over a dozen drugs for these seniors to take every day is not uncommon. Reports of some seniors taking over two dozen or more drugs exist.

Although during recent years, a movement of deprescribing (rational use of drugs by eliminating unnecessary ones) has started, we are still dealing with the same type of synthetic drugs. These drugs had no prior contact with the human body and were only being approved after preliminary testing that showed they hadn't caused us serious harm in the short period of a decade or two of clinical trials. But they are still unproven long-term. The real test of their validity in treating any disease with their inevitable accompanying side-effects, toxicity, or safety, after entering our complex body, has only begun. Only experience over time will find out whether or not they are indeed safe or suitable for a particular illness, with their side-effects simultaneously being treated by more drugs. This has been common in the practice of modern medicine for decades. It is no different from the budding phase of the practice of Chinese medicine millennia ago. The former (after approval through clinical trials) are still in the early trial-and-error stage of testing, while the latter had already done it thousands of years earlier. Why do we want to do the same with brand-new synthetic chemicals now, and begin anew to try to find out whether or not they are safe or really work, long-term? Do we really want to wait another thousand years (or even 2000 years) to find out?

We can't afford to continue the current vicious cycle of toxic drugs beget new diseases that in turn require more toxic drugs to counter. We need true preventive healthcare and true herbal supplements and more tried-and-true non-synthetic and less-toxic drugs. These can complement other modern drugs by ameliorating their toxic side-effects to help make Americans naturally healthier. Just consider what these synthetic drugs and chemicals have done to our environment and to our body in a period of only seventy of my conscious years. We still continue to use them with abandon. I believe the increasing cancer incidences are partly due to the toxic chemicals and drugs now ubiquitously present on our planet. At the same time, our environment is now rendered so germ-free with antibiotics that if you want to buy a plain soap without antibiotics, you'll have to look hard unless you know the exact brand. Hand sanitizers are everywhere. Meat from antibiotic-fed animals is common. Yet the current medical wisdom is only to wash your hands often in a flu epidemic, which is fine if you simply use soap without antibiotics. Soaps with antibiotics help to contribute to the weakening of our resistance to infectious diseases. Even in this day and age, when you get a cold and are scared enough by the medical or pharmaceutical establishment's teachings, and go to see a doctor, chances are he/she would prescribe an antibiotic without doing any bacterial culture, just in case the cough may turn into pneumonia. Imagine what the oral antibiotics would do to the beneficial bacteria in your gut. These microbes (including fungi and viruses), known as microbiome, have been with us since the dawn of human history. They have played a crucial role in our health and wellbeing throughout our human history. I have personally witnessed the progression of the loss (or weakening) of our resistance to diseases (immunity) during the past seventy years. I suspect Crohn's disease and many other now-common gastrointestinal illnesses are due to the indiscriminate use of antibiotics and the weakening of our immune system by some of our modern lifestyles.

Only recently have scientists started to realize the importance of our microbiome for our wellbeing and to find non-drug ways to deal with these diseases.

All the above affect your health and I hope you will agree with me after reading the rest of this chapter.

INAPPROPRIATE OR FAUX SCIENCE – WHERE LIES THE TRUTH?

There is one thing fundamentally wrong with drugs and herbal supplements. It's our <u>failure</u> to consider <u>both</u> the therapeutic entity and our body that ingests it, <u>together</u>. The therapeutic entity can be either a chemical drug or a complex herbal medicine that interacts with our infinitely complex living body. What follows describes the therapeutic entity (drug or herb) and its inevitable interactions with our body which ultimately will lead to our wellbeing or demise:

1. In the <u>development</u> and <u>quality control</u> of drugs, there is no problem using advanced scientific technologies to achieve both. But with herbal supplements, the scientific technologies used to analyze them have been inappropriate since these products were first introduced after the passage of the Dietary Supplement Health and Education Act (DSHEA) in 1994. The appropriate analyses for complex herbal materials (true herbal supplements) had not yet been developed. So, due to misunderstanding, human inertia, and expediency, the scientists involved simply used the technologies already developed specifically for pure-chemical drugs on these herbs. They seemed to have forgotten to consider that these technologies might not work for herbs that are undefined complex mixtures of many chemicals

as opposed to drugs that are clearly identified and well-defined chemicals, often appearing as a single chemical when used as modern drugs. Up to this day, an herb like 'Echinacea' is still analytically viewed only as a single-chemical entity such as its chlorogenic acid (one of its myriad of chemicals) as a marker for its identity and quality. This same chemical can be equally used as an identity- and quality-marker for honeysuckle herb and coffee extracts because it is also present in both in sizable quantities. There lies the persistent problem. Commercial 'herbal' supplements containing this easily analyzable marker (chlorogenic acid) could be labeled 'Echinacea,' 'honeysuckle,' or 'coffee' supplement and legally sold as 'herbal' supplements, standardized to a certain amount of this chemical. Incidentally, one of my fellow pharmacognosists and good friend, Alvin Segelman, PhD, (used to be a professor at Rutgers University and later Director of R&D at Nature's Sunshine before he retired) once did an experiment to illustrate this controversial point. Al made an extract of Echinacea and standardized it to its chlorogenic acid (polyphenolics) content. He then made an extract of dried horse manure and added a comparable analyzable amount of chlorogenic acid (a polyphenol) to it, plus some inert carriers to make it look like an herbal product. He labeled the product 'Echinacea.' Since they were both 'standardized' to the same amount of polyphenols (analyzed as chlorogenic acid), no one could tell the difference because analytical chemists only tested them for the content of the standardized chemical(s) while the other parts of the product could be anything. [see **Chapter 9: Adulteration Continues...** and **LCHN-13**]

2. Our body is not the visual single entity we normally see. It is an extremely complex organism containing countless chemicals, cells, tissues and other matters, but never a single variable, nor can it be turned into one. Nothing we do can change that fact. When it comes to putting drugs in our body, no science can help you other than to keep trying them one after another until one works better than the others and with fewer side effects. When

a new drug is approved by our FDA to be used for a certain disease, there is no guarantee it will work for you. Neither the pharmacist nor the doctor can guarantee you. You have no choice but to trust their word and recommendation. They in turn get their knowledge on the drug from the pharmaceutical industry (e.g., publications, announcements, or its salespeople). The ultimate information still has to come from more trial and error over time in humans, be it months, years, decades, centuries, or longer. Thus, even though the drug development part may be scientific, once the drug enters the human body composed of multiple variables, it is just trial and error as our ancestors had done millennia ago with herbs. That's why there is the traditional wisdom that practice of medicine is an art, referring to the traditional ancient medicine, not what we now have which we call modern medicine. Only during recent decades have we started to call modern medicine 'scientific' while referring to ancient traditional medicine as witchcraft or art. But neither is scientific. Anything we do relating to our body as a whole is a virtual mess. If you doubt that, just ask yourself why the drug companies still have not come up with safer and better-performing drugs after sixty to seventy years of trying. Instead, their drugs are mostly toxic and don't work well. Every time a drug is introduced into our body, there is no guarantee it will work as we have wanted or planned it to, without causing side-effects. In any other industries that produce, and claim to have products like drug therapy with so many basic defective parts, I think they would be bankrupt in no time. But the Pharmaceutical Industrial Complex (PIC: including drug makers, marketers, insurance companies, politicians, and anyone financially associated with, or indebted, to drug companies) have been thriving! We, as Americans, have given them all the incentives to continue to produce these drugs because we somehow have continued to condone what they are doing and pay whatever they demand, at least so far. Thus, they have no incentive to change anything for our benefit but to continue to produce more toxic drugs and collect income with apparently no liabilities. That's why we have our current *status quo* – American culture of drugs and more drugs. We are now so entrenched in this culture that we need these toxic drugs, many of which are used for countering the side-effects of drug-caused diseases. Nothing can change for the short term.

Meanwhile, I believe the PIC continues to have an outsize role in our national health care. They have done an excellent job so far for themselves by quashing competition and holding American consumers hostage. They do so by affording us no alternative to their toxic drugs. Their overwhelmingly strong technological influence on the scientists working on the only potential alternative (i.e., herbal supplements) over the past decades has brought us to our current state. Misapplying pharmaceutical technologies specifically developed for chemical drugs on complex herbs has generated wrong or ambiguous results, hence much controversy. These in turn have caused most scientists to view herbs from the wrong perspective, based on ambiguous or invalid data, without even being aware of the basic differences of chemicals versus herbs (or food) that have been causing these problems.

Here is an example of how inappropriate science is used. In drug testing, such as trying to determine the aspirin content in tablets of different aspirin formulations, we use pure aspirin as our standard and analyze the different brands one at a time to determine how much aspirin is present in each. That is done one brand at a time. It is standard science. However, after we have done Brand A, we want to do more brands, adding Brands B and C, for example. But now, to expedite the process, we don't want to do them one at a time. We want to analyze them all at once - samples of A, B and C thrown together. We could do that, but we wouldn't get the same correct results because there is no other appropriate technology to do all samples mixed together all at once and get appropriate results for each product. You may use educated or wild guesses to arrive at some result or numbers. But then, that's not science; it's more like gambling. And this is what happens in the field of our herbal supplement development process and their usage in humans. Alternatively, you could use machines that can analyze each brand of aspirin simultaneously side by side using the same standard. But you can't throw all the brands together and analyze them that way. At least with drugs like aspirin, the standard (reference) is a single entity; and aspirin is aspirin. With herbs, the standard is not a single entity, nor is the material (sample) to be tested. Both are a multi-chemical mess. You can't just take a bell-shaped fruit and analyze it for pectin and Vitamin C amongst hundreds or thousands of other chemicals and decide to call either chemical a pear. Nor can you pick and analyze chlorogenic acid in Echinacea and call that chemical Echinacea.

Although the above drug testing belongs in the realm of chemical science, I believe its basic scientific principle is still the same for other sciences such as biological, physiological, and pharmacological – the aim is to compare a standard (constant) with test samples (variables) one at a time to see the differences. However, after encountering so many discrepancies over my 55 years of experience in the sciences of natural products, especially during the past twenty years, I have started to have doubts whether or not there is still scientific integrity or truth in this confusing, self-serving, market- and money-driven world. Scientific truth has increasingly been twisted to fit one's agenda to arrive at the current drug therapy dilemma. The toxic drugs produced by the existing pharmaceutical system cause new diseases (e.g., tardive dyskinesia) that require more new toxic drugs (e.g., valbenazine) to treat, in a never-ending vicious cycle. We have to pay for all of these disease-generating toxic drugs and then for the drugs to treat diseases they have caused. Yet drug makers and marketers continue to make money on us with apparent impunity. I have tried for at least twenty years to persuade my expert colleagues in government, industry, and academia to address this issue, but so far not a single one in government or academia has even openly acknowledged such a problem exists. When I speak openly on this topic, some in industry and academia consider me a trouble maker, though nobody has ever called me a liar. Once, I overheard a discussion of the truth relating to some Chinese herb topic involving me, someone said, "If Al Leung thinks it's correct, it is fine with me." I considered that quite a compliment. But I don't remember who she was. [See **Introduction** and relevant topics in **LCHN**]

Regarding my outspoken opinions on drugs and herbs, some of my colleagues and friends in government and industry may know they should do something but their hands are tied. Others are so drowned in their position and self-importance that they never even understand (or try to understand) the overall issues. This has led to my decision to simultaneously republish **LCHN** and publish my **Memoir** to try to bring my story to you, the American public and consumers. You don't need to be technical or have an advanced degree to understand what I am trying to say. All you need is your common sense.

For the sake of our children, grandchildren, and theirs, I feel obliged to sound the alarm to the general public, so that it may be aware of what has been happening in a major part of our life, which is healthcare, and more specifically, <u>expensive toxic drugs</u> and <u>often worthless alternatives</u>.

THE DRUG

Scientifically, the drug itself (usually a chemical) is the least problem. It can be synthesized or isolated from nature and can be uniquely identified and analyzed without being confused with other chemicals. If it is synthetic, it is basically brand new to our planet, with no prior association with any living organisms on earth like plants, animals, microbes, and humans. And its actions on these living organisms are totally unknown. Hence, turning it into a drug for treating human illnesses is like throwing darts at a target, blindfolded. Since we have not the slightest clue what this new chemical can do, we design all sorts of 'scientific' hypotheses to find out. To test whether or not it can do a particular job, we have to make all kinds of assumptions and test it in test tubes, cells, and then in animals before subjecting the drug to human testing. During all this testing, most chemicals never make it through the initial stages. The few that have succeeded in going through these tests and clinical trials may then be approved for human use. However, it is only then that the real testing begins, and with uncertainty, like trial and error. Unlike traditional herbal medicines with millennia of human-use history, this new drug has none; and its true human-use experience only starts now, after being approved for human use. New synthetic drugs like this have <u>at most</u> 100 years of human contact except for a few natural ones like morphine and ephedrine that were isolated from nature years earlier.

But then, their synthetic sister drugs are the ones with which we have so many problems nowadays, including opioids and amphetamines.

Although chemically easy to define, our modern drugs have been, for decades, developed using sciences that offer no provisions to deal with the chaos encountered as soon as they enter the human body to supposedly take care of whatever makes it sick by neutralizing the presumed targeted culprit(s). To us intelligent humans, we know our body is infinitely complex and simultaneously well organized. But to a lifeless pure chemical drug entering our body, there is <u>no direction from an all-knowing being</u> (certainly not any scientist or medical doctor) to lead it directly to where we think the cause of our ailment is and to neutralize it. The presumed causative agent targeted can be a chemical such as a specific receptor or enzyme, any cell content, cell structure, or a myriad of other entities that make up our body. Yet we expect this developed drug to somehow navigate itself to one or two specific entities in our body to do its job without bumping into countless other moving targets to cause havoc in our body? And how are we sure whatever the targeted culprits are actually <u>the</u> ones? We simply don't know! Something is not right with this picture. I don't recognize the science there, and I'm a legitimate, upstanding scientist not without accomplishments. Yet I had been unaware of this for decades before my epiphany about 15 years ago! One thing we can call this kind of human activity is – gambling! If you don't agree, I would like a legitimate, free-thinking scientist to tell us otherwise in an understandable language. When such a scientist, indebted to no one, appears, maybe he/she can also tell us why we have spent seventy plus years and billions and billions of dollars in developing scientific drugs yet we still can't have decent nontoxic ones that work, without causing hidden diseases that would haunt us when we get older. In the meantime, more and more new diseases keep popping up. And we continue to spend money on these toxic drugs, whether we like it or not. I think it would be an eye-opener to find out how many new diseases have been caused by toxic drugs since 1980 and the amount of money and effort spent in countering them. I wonder who would have the courage and money to do this kind of research. I believe the underlying cause is not the drugs themselves, but our extremely complex living body when the drugs enter it to interact with it!

Furthermore, these synthetic drugs are now ubiquitous in our environment; and I'm not even talking about agricultural chemicals! Some of the drugs are flushed down the toilet or discarded in dumps unused, while others are sent there as metabolites through our body wastes. Considering so many people take up to a dozen or more drugs per day and the pharmaceutical industry keeps producing more and more in number and in quantity to take advantage of this self-generated demand, the toxin load due to drugs in our environment must be sizable. I believe that all these are sitting on our earth like a time bomb waiting quietly for our descendants to deal with, much like toxic wastes from other manufacturing processes, but much more widely distributed throughout our earth.

THE HERBAL SUPPLEMENT

At first glance, the scientific situation is much worse with herbal products. Instead of a single constant as with a known chemical drug, we now have a so-called constant of an herb or formula consisting of multiple chemicals (both known and unknown), which hardly can be considered a constant (except maybe visually). When we introduce this herbal supplement into our complex body, we will have total chaos. However, if treated correctly, the situation can be turned in our favor because our body has co-evolved with all of the chemicals in this herbal mix since antiquity. Herbs are like foods, we have personal experience with them for millennia. We have also already inherited the knowledge to tell which is edible or not toxic, and which kills. Therefore, there is no need to start testing them from scratch as with synthetic drugs. The key is to consider them as foods, as the DSHEA had originally intended when it was passed in 1994. However, chemists right from the start have been treating them as drugs or pure chemicals because they didn't know better. That is the root of most of our problems with herbal supplements.

Nevertheless, the chemicals in herbs are not brand-new chemicals like synthetics that all of a sudden appear on our planet. These natural chemicals simply return to earth from where they have come. Hence, I believe there is no time bomb there for our posterity.

OUR COMPLEX BODY

Depending on our faiths and beliefs, we somehow have been given, or evolved into, an extremely complex body with all its chemicals, cells, tissues, and organs working independently and together in miraculous efficiency. We'd never be able to figure out how exactly it works and how to fix it whenever it breaks down, especially physiologically and mentally; and we'll die trying. It would be easier to build a human-like robot from scratch and fix whatever breaks down than trying to tamper with our body that already has everything perfectly in place and is functioning well despite some rare exceptions. Any major disturbance anywhere in our body is going to affect its other parts. The ramifications can be diseases or general malaise.

Over the past several millennia, the Chinese have developed the *yin* & *yang* concept to try to deal with this. Thus, we are well when the *yin* & *yang* in our body are balanced; and when they are off balance, we become ill. Though we don't know exactly what they are. Many things cause imbalance such as stress, toxic effects of drugs, and excessive physical activities, among others. There are herbs that help to restore this balance, especially the tonic herbs. The introduction of a new foreign chemical (e.g., a synthetic drug) into our body, which can go everywhere inside us trying to do its job (whatever that may be) is bound to cause a serious disturbance. This basic flaw in our drug therapy process might have started simply as a case of negligence or misunderstanding on the part of the scientists involved. They might have had originally developed the processes about 100 years ago but had forgotten (or might not have had even realized) that our body is a complex system with a myriad of living and moving materials and not simply an easily visible single entity. At the time, when the drug development and drug therapy processes were forming (> 100 years ago), it is understandable humans and plants could be physically seen as single entities and treated as such. Consequently, these processes have since been followed and enabled by other scientists, including myself, up until fifteen or so years ago. When it concerns drugs, we all have, at one time or another, without thinking, accepted our body as a single entity and not as a complex system with countless variables. So, when something like a drug gets into our body, we used to think it would deal with a single entity, but in reality, it meets instant chaos instead.

OUR BODY MEETS THE DRUG – IRREDEEMABLE CHAOS

When a brand-new modern synthetic drug enters our body, we have no idea how our body would react to this foreign object. Furthermore, your body is different from mine. Hence, your guess is as good as mine trying to predict how our bodies would react. One thing we may be sure is that our body would have no historical or innate memory of this new chemical. Only time would help our body to get over the initial shock and eventually get used to its presence and learn to live with it, provided it would not have killed us by then. That may be centuries or millennia. For now, there is nothing we can do but grin and bear it and at the same time try to reset our thinking about drug therapy.

When this kind of new drug enters our body, it meets chaos. This chaos cannot be resolved, due to the nature of the new drug. If it is synthetic, it is brand new to our planet. It may harm and pollute. Even if you could turn our bodies into a single-entity variable, you could not erase the fact that this new drug has never been tested in humans for more than a period of ten to twenty years (the time a clinical trial may take) before it is approved. Hence, its safety in humans over time is still totally unknown. In another few decades or centuries of use, some totally unexpected effects may still start showing up, good or bad.

OUR BODY MEETS THE HERBAL SUPPLEMENT — REDEEMABLE CHAOS

As I have explained earlier, herbal supplements are more complex than a chemical drug, because compared to drugs they have countless chemicals. When they enter the body to meet its contents, it is not just one item interacting with chaos (our body) as with drugs. It is itself chaos that meets more chaos to give us total chaos. Fortunately, herbs have one thing in their favor. Like foods, they have evolved with our body since ancient times, so our body has knowledge of them. Along with their detailed documented records (esp. Chinese and Indian herbs), we know which herbs/formulas are safe and which can be rendered safe or are inherently toxic. So there is no need of testing from scratch as with pure chemicals, especially synthetic ones. Using <u>appropriate</u> scientific technologies, we can make modern naturally derived drugs and current herbal supplements safer. But we have to treat herbs as foods rather than as drugs, as DSHEA rightly suggested when it was passed over twenty years ago.

About seventeen years ago (2001), my company, Phyto-Technologies, Inc., was awarded a Small Business Innovation Research (SBIR) grant of around $1.4 million for determining the antimigraine ingredients of feverfew for clinical trial. It took five years to complete the project. But we couldn't find any institution or money to do the clinical trial thereafter, so the project results have remained unused. However, out of this research, we did develop a system to handle complex herbs so that they can be scientifically and correctly analyzed with consistent and reproducible results. We called this system Phyto-True. From now on, we won't have to treat herbs assuming they only contain one or two specific known compounds that are responsible for all of the herbs' properties. However, the rest of the world's practitioners have not started the proper scientific approach yet, because most scientists still think the chemical-specific drug technologies are 'scientific' and therefore are still widely used. But, honestly, how scientific is it when you arbitrarily choose and assign one or two active chemical compounds to an herb, among many others also present (e.g., those with anti-inflammatory, antioxidant, laxative, anti-tumor, anti-viral, narcotic, or psychotropic activities), and call these your <u>marker(s) of identity and quality for that herb</u>? Many times the ones you have selected have no relevance to what the herb is traditionally used for. Take feverfew, for example. Its leaves have been traditionally used for preventing migraine for generations in Europe. Three clinical trials had been performed with raw or freeze-dried leaves and had positive results. Around 2000, our National Institutes of Health (NIH) either was planning to support or had been supporting such a clinical trial when another report from a clinical trial in the Netherlands using a feverfew extract with a marker chemical (parthenolide) in high concentration (0.35%) yielded negative results. This marker chemical had been widely assumed (and still is assumed) to be the active principle of feverfew. That was when NIH abandoned the project and issued a Small Business Innovation Research (SBIR) request for proposal (RFP) for small businesses (companies with less than 200 employees) to send in their proposals. Mine, not fixated on any known chemical(s) but based on fingerprinting different extracts/fractions and comparing with those from plants used in a positive trial done earlier in England, was awarded the SBIR grant. Our research showed that parthenolide by itself would have no antimigraine activity. This activity resides in an oil-soluble fraction of feverfew. So, this is just one example to show the fallacy of assuming one or two known chemicals to represent the total active properties of herbs.

Also, don't forget the horse manure example described earlier. Incidentally, our Phyto-True fingerprinting would have no problem telling which is the real echinacea product and which is the horse manure one.

Our Phyto-True system is by no means a tried-and-true technology yet, but it can be used as the first step in properly handling complex Chinese herbs to retain their traditional properties. With this new technology, we can start producing some true alternatives to chemical drugs. I wish to thank my team that included Dennis Awang, Greg Pennyroyal, Allison McCutcheon, Chin-Fu Chen, Heather Conway, Shannon Ehlers, and Darin Smith for their efforts, without them this technology would not have been developed. Furthermore, my sincere thanks go to NCCAM for the grant, and the reviewers of our proposal, one of whom I later found out to be Frank Jaksch, the founder of Chromadex. A special thank goes to Marguerite Klein, our program officer, for her championing of our project. I also want to thank Karriem Ali (aka Karyem Allife), Marilyn Barrett, and Ezra Bejar for their input; they had earlier been co-members with me on Leiner's Botanical Science Board.

There are over 12,000 Chinese herbs and more than 130,000 herbal formulas documented in the Chinese herbal medicine (CHM) literature during a period of about 3,500 years. I have often written about this in my **LCHN** and other publications. Unfortunately, in recent decades, due to the strong influence of the pharmaceutical industry, the Chinese scientists have been actually 'modernizing' CHM based on the assumed-active-chemical concept, discarding tradition as nonscientific and adopting faux science as the real thing. Because of this, during the past sixteen or seventeen years, CHM has become so commercialized that even one of the most well-known Chinese tonics, cured fo-ti (*zhiheshouwu*) has now become a chemical source for a sister chemical of resveratrol called 2,3,5,4'-tetrahydroxystilbene glucoside (THSG). In the short span of two decades, cured fo-ti has changed its traditional character. Rather than using it in its original form that had been used for over a thousand years, now it's turned into a 'fo-ti' that contains the strong antioxidant chemical, THSG, whether or not it is in the raw (toxic, laxative) or cured (antiaging tonic) form. This chemical is currently in vogue because it is one of the strong antioxidants like resveratrol. It was not even present in any significant amount in the original, traditionally cured fo-ti; and it should be only present in the raw fo-ti that is traditionally considered toxic as well as a laxative. Many of the current herbal supplements are not really herbal as the New York Attorney General already discovered earlier in 2015. [see **Chapter 13: Proper Modernization...**]

WHAT CAN WE DO WITH THE DRUGS?

Unfortunately, the drug situation has been so entrenched that there is nothing straight-forward that can be done. However, the general public needs to understand that the practice of medicine (esp. internal and general) has never been totally scientific. It is not like some part of surgery and dentistry where damaged body parts can be replaced with 'bionic' parts with more and more precision. In that area, examples abound, including implant lenses, teeth, and other replaced body parts. Even there, it's not all science. Skill and experience are essential, and there remains the possibility of rejection. Hence, practice of medicine has always been a mixture of art and science. Now, at an advanced age, I have finally found out why. When drugs or herbs enter our body, there is no real science there – faux science, perhaps. The drugs may be scientifically developed, but when they enter our complex body, they meet chaos. Hence, an experienced and skillful physician would be a much better doctor than one whose experience is limited to following the promotional literature of the pharmaceutical industry. In drug therapy, only the drug part is scientific. Once it enters the body to treat an illness, it is just the physician's experience, skill, and the art of trial and error; and only time will tell. Yet for decades, it has been claimed to be scientific, despite the fact that the drugs are simply being subjected to trial and error. This produces unpredictable results, often with side-effects some of which have since become new diseases.

WHAT CAN WE DO WITH HERBAL SUPPLEMENTS?

Compared to drugs, herbal supplements are a very minor part of our healthcare expenditures – tens of billions of dollars versus hundreds of billions to trillions with drugs. Drugs are a large part of our national health care; and heath care consumes a major part of our government's and our own financial resources. We can't do much about drugs for now but we certainly can do something immediately about herbs. There are two ways to go about it. One is to improve the current so-called herbal supplements on the market which are mostly chemicals or drugs disguised as herbal supplements. The other is to bring well-known CHM formulas in a truly modernized form to the modern world using <u>appropriate</u> scientific technologies, starting with Phyto-True, the concept and technology described earlier.

Except for a period when I had hay fever in graduate school in Michigan and some years afterwards in New Jersey (which I got rid of when I discovered the treatment with magnolia flower buds), I seldom have been sick in all my life. But when I do, I have several Chinese formulas made in China handy which I use for colds, flus, stomach troubles, coughs, pimples, and canker sores, among others. My family also uses them and I sometimes give them to friends when they need them. They are much better (and safer) than most of the over-the-counter drugs on the market.

Getting rid of fake herbal supplements to be sure consumers are taking the real ones will save them money and will prevent possible deleterious effects due to their taking mere new chemicals with inert carriers. Herbs and formulas have been used for not decades but centuries or millennia. From our ancestors' experience up to the present, we already know what herbs or formulas to avoid so that the ones we have now have already been vetted over time. Their toxic or beneficial nature at least is known for us to decide whether or not to use them. But that is not true with specific chemicals in the herbs. In large doses, they are basically being used out of context. Their safety is not known. It is like new synthetic drugs going through human testing all over again. Their only difference from synthetics is that they have been (evolved) with us for a long time in small quantities. But in large doses? They still have to be used with caution! Furthermore, once the natural ones are synthesized, they are no longer the same, unless we can assure their purity to be at least 100.00%, containing not even 0.01% impurities. Remember the synthetic analgesic W-18 being 10,000 times stronger than morphine described earlier? Even a 'fairy-dust' amount of this or a similar strong synthetic chemical present in the impurity of the synthetic counterpart of your natural chemical could spell trouble.

Despite all these issues, genuine herbal supplements will save consumers a lot of money because they will no longer throw away their money and get nothing in return. Instead, they will get true health benefits. Furthermore, those who need modern drugs can still continue to get them; but I believe they would now use them with more caution, after knowing the myth of drugs being 'scientific' and herbs 'nonscientific.'

I can envision a new natural drug industry built around modernized herbs and formulas for the benefits of consumers who need help with their health care but are already wary of modern toxic drugs. This new industry can be funded by consumers and others who truly believe in helping their neighbors while themselves also benefiting from their own kindness to others. With the power and efficiency of the Internet, the first company that will serve as a prototype of this new industry, can be organized with the support of consumers to sell true herbal products already being sold under DSHEA as herbal supplements. The next step would be selling natural drugs, currently being sold as dietary supplements or disguised as 'herbal' supplements. These new drugs include huperzine A, resveratrol, THSG, berberine, and lutein, among many others, which show promise for different conditions. They can be manufactured and sold at minimum markups (e.g., 5-10%) instead of the usual 100% to 1,000% (or higher) markups as commonly practiced by herbal product purveyors, while drug companies will charge any price they want, supposedly to justify recovering their development and patent costs.

The new companies could be a consumer-funded or nonprofit type of organization to produce more effective and safer herbal supplements at a fraction of the cost of most OTC drugs. No one should be allowed to prey on the poor health of fellow-humans to shamelessly enrich themselves and get away with it. If shaming pharmaceutical companies and 'herbal'-supplement marketers doesn't work, taking part of their business away may.

CHAPTER 13

Proper Modernization of Chinese Medicine

As I said earlier in the chapter on my **Growing up in Asia**, I was raised in a traditional Chinese medical environment and grew up using Chinese herbs. My maternal great grandfather was a village doctor and I was told that he treated village patients the typical traditional way as in bygone days, with compassion and received whatever they could afford to pay him. He lived to be over 80 years old.

I believe my grandmother gained her knowledge of using herbs from him, since she married into the family when she was only around 15, as was common in those days, and there were no schools for women to learn these things. All the years while my sisters and I were growing up, my grandma was our family doctor. I don't remember ever visiting any modern doctors until our twin sisters were about four years old (and I was around twelve) when the older twin (we called her Big Twin) had scarlet fever. I had to carry her on my back (in a piggyback ride) down from our terrace more than a hundred steps down to the main street at sea level to take the bus to go to a hospital. She was given antibiotics that must have been some form of penicillin because that was the first miracle drug available. But my grandma got the permission of the Western doctor (a Chinese) to use American ginseng on Big Twin to lower her fever and to keep her system cool. That was my first real experience with Western medicine, successfully used along with Chinese medicine. I never knew my maternal grandfather until I was in my preteen years after he returned home from Cuba. Even after that, I barely saw him, not to speak of having a regular grandfather. But he must have also learned enough TCM practices (including herbs) from my great grandfather before he left for Cuba when he was in his late teens. Otherwise how would he have happened to own an herb shop among the three of his businesses? When my wife and I visited Cuba on a 'study' trip in 2003 with the American Museum of Natural History, I actually visited his herb shop in Havana.

In any case, as I have grown up in that kind of tradition, especially using herbs, I always had a wish of helping people as my great grandfather did. And it was also my intention to be a doctor to help others.

I distinctly remember one occasion long ago, must be in the 1970's, when my brother-in-law (Nelson Thayer, a Yale-in-China scholar) was still alive. For some reason, I got hold of an article from Yale University related to its work in China, probably from Nelson. It was a report written by an MD professor. There was a segment dealing with Chinese healthcare workers. The author lamented on the conditions under which Chinese doctors were working, especially their status and salaries. He reported that those needed to be improved because they were way below our American standards. I don't remember much about the rest of that report. Nor do I remember whether or not he also suggested improving the general standard of living of the Chinese population at the time. However, one thought has since stuck in my mind. I believe the Chinese doctors at the time were not there for making a lot of money; they just wanted to do their job helping others who were living not that much below their own standard of living, maybe half or one-third. But unlike in the United States, the income gap between doctors practicing in affluent areas and patients in poor areas can be five to ten or twenty times more. I didn't know what doctors made in the US at that time, compared to the average income of American patients. But I thought it odd that a Western doctor should consider the Chinese doctors to be above their own people, coming down from their high station to treat the lowly peasants. I believe my great grandfather was not like that, nor the Chinese doctors in the 1970's. They were all living in the same village, town, or nearby. The doctors were just doing their job. High salaries and status were not what they would seek. In any case, for the first time, I got a glimpse of how doctors in the United States might consider their practice of medicine. It was not just about helping people, but also about money and power. At the time, I found it disappointing. But it was just the beginning of my learning about health care in the USA. It is complicated and controlled by a few interdependent powerful interests. The reason I was trying to get into medical school was because I wanted to help others as my great grandfather did. Money and status never entered my mind. Obviously, what I was aspiring to do was not conventional doctoring. Perhaps that Yale doctor was ahead of his times in caring about status and prestige, as it has become more common now in the USA. Although I never studied conventional medicine, what I have been doing with Chinese herbal medicine has touched many more people and benefitted their health more than if I had become a medical doctor. Now, I want to let the general public know about the *status quo* of drugs and herbal supplements and suggest a fundamental way to change it. Instead of toxic drugs, we can have a true herbal alternative to benefit many more people than synthetic drugs. At the same time, it would cause them much less pain and misery. [See **Chapter 1: Growing up in Asia** and **Chapter 14: What should we do...**]

Anyhow, because of my weakness in math after skipping my junior year of high school, my total grade on the entrance exams to the National Taiwan University was not high enough to get me assigned to study medicine. To qualify to study medicine at that time, one probably needed to score one of the highest grades in the entrance exams. Consequently, for the first year, I studied geology; and for the second year, I had to take the entrance exams again and this time I was assigned to pharmacy. But that was close enough for me. It had somehow turned out to be almost what I had exactly needed to do to follow my great grandfather's footsteps.

During my four years in Pharmacy School in NTU, I was interested in Chinese materia medica (literally, medical materials) or *sheng yao* that means 'crude drugs' or raw herbs in Chinese. That is more or less the same as pharmacognosy in the West, except the drugs are all Chinese medicines from different sources including animals and minerals, which, for convenience, are all simply called herbs. Nevertheless, we did use Heber Youngken's *Textbook of Pharmacognosy* for learning the scientific basics. I did well in it and was offered a teaching assistantship to pursue graduate studies at the University of Michigan. Somehow in my undergraduate studies and later in graduate school, I was directed steadily towards the identification and isolation of the active principles (see **Glossary**) of plant drugs, always searching for that chemical that is believed to be responsible for most of the activities known for a particular herb. For years, like my fellow students and later my colleagues, I never questioned the Western wisdom on this, until about only 15 years ago. Then, I started to realize that the Western approach to herbs was nothing but seeking chemical drugs from herbs, trying to replace herbs with modern drugs.

This Western approach is not making use of the millennia-old documented record of Chinese medicines' human experience and wisdom that are not built in days, weeks, years, or even decades, but in centuries and millennia. These experiences and wisdom have kept the Chinese people alive and healthy for thousands of years. The current continuing call for modernization (basically westernization) has been misleading. It is, in fact, anything, but modernization. The term 'pharmaceuticalization' would be more appropriate, since once any chemical is isolated from the herb, it doesn't represent the herb anymore, nor does it have the long-documented total attributes of the herb to represent its properties and functions. Hence, no matter how you call this chemical or group of chemicals, it is neither traditional herbal medicine nor modernized herbal medicine. It is a chemical drug, even though it may not be a synthetic one.

During the past century, we put aside the traditional experience and wisdom of Chinese herbs, and have persisted in pursuing a completely different type of therapeutics based on brand-new synthetic chemicals. These chemicals have no prior presence in our environment, hence no human experience whatsoever; thus, their toxicity and safety for humans are totally unknown. The results from drug development and drug therapy efforts over the past seven or eight decades have consistently produced deleterious effects in those humans who have taken these drugs. These modern and scientifically produced drugs have continued to produce side effects some of which end up causing new diseases that require more such drugs to treat and the vicious cycle continues.

This vicious cycle was officially started by the FDA's approval of the allegedly first drug valbenazine on April 11, 2017, for treating a new disease called tardive dyskinesia (delayed uncontrollable body movements) caused by the use of antipsychotic, anti-epilepsy, and gastrointestinal drugs over the course of several decades. Incidentally, the marketer of this new drug set its price at $64,000 - $128,000 per patient per year, or $175 - $350 per day (40mg/80mg daily)! Like all modern drugs, valbenazine was already listed to have numerous side-effects, some of which can be dangerous and are bound to produce more new diseases.

All this happens because our body is extremely complex, and these synthetic chemicals or modified natural chemicals have had no history interacting with it. It would take them more than just decades before their true nature will be known.

As many of us know, herbs are just like foods. There is no one single chemical in any herb (or food) which has all the properties of the herb. As I have written many times before and elsewhere in this **Memoir** and in the republished **LCHN**, pectin (present in apple) cannot be called an apple, nor can a ginsenoside in ginseng or in a Chinese gourd (*jiaogulan*) be called ginseng.

Since isolating a chemical from an herb to represent its totality is impossible, it ends up that any chemical from that herb with any kind of activity which could be turned into a drug would do for the natural product scientists seeking drugs from herbs. But these chemicals don't represent the herbs in most cases. It only means that we have found some chemical we think we need but which has nothing to do with the herb's documented attributes. The end result is we have not utilized the traditional wisdom and experience we have of the herbs. Instead, the *status quo* of close to 100 years is maintained, synthesizing sister compounds to imitate a natural one (e.g., morphine) to get an ever faster-acting and stronger one to replace the natural one. This is not what Nature has meant to provide us.

Some herbs do yield active principles responsible for most of their intended actions. An example is Mexican magic mushrooms, such as *Psilocybe* species, which yield psilocybin that has been proven hallucinogenic. I suspect the two closely related ones I isolated from *Psilocybe baeocystis* during my graduate school years, are also active as hallucinogens, which I named baeocystin and norbaeocystin. However, the vast majority of Chinese herbs don't have one or two chemicals in them that account for their 'total' effects. Whatever properties they have (most of which are documented) don't reside in one or two chemicals, but rather, in many of the chemicals present in the herbs, working together to perform their traditionally known and documented actions.

All through those years and many thereafter, I was always thinking 'active principles' as everybody else, putting true herbs in some corner deep in my mind. When herbal supplements came along in the early 1990's, it took me another 10 years or so to start questioning the logic of <u>herbal supplements being treated as drugs while legally classified as food.</u> Then it dawned on me that we never had to deal with this dilemma before. We had always treated drugs as drugs and herbs also as drugs (i.e., their active chemicals or active principles that we seek) and never had to deal with the original nature of the herbs. But suddenly we had herbal supplements that are regulated as foods. What should we do with them?

When this whole herbal supplement thing started, we had no scientific technologies to deal with these complex herbs as they have been known and documented over centuries. So we treated them right away as drugs (chemicals), not so much as active principles, but simply as active chemicals or marker compounds that might have no relevance to the action of the herbs concerned. We have since held these complex herbs to the standards set for drugs. Seriously, apple, ginseng, raisin, Echinacea, and goji as drugs, to be treated and analyzed just as a drug like aspirin? Or should they be treated appropriately as herbal supplements? You would think by now, over 20 years after DSHEA was passed, we would have noticed our folly from the erratic results we have so far obtained from research on herbs all these years. No, we are still actively doing the same thing over and over. However, we now have the basics we call Phyto-True technologies to start dealing with herbs properly. It is only a tiny step in the right direction towards true herbal supplements or genuine herbal products. But this step must be taken to extract ourselves from the hold of toxic synthetic drugs on our healthcare.

The general idea is that there are better ways to look at herbs. Instead of simply treating them as drugs to make them fit our preconceived drug concepts, we should start looking at herbs as foods, or closer to foods. The logic of our current treatment of herbs is no different than taking a food like apple and insisting on analyzing it specifically for its pectin (among a myriad of its other phytochemicals) and consider pectin, apple, or analyze an herb like 'Echinacea' for a phenolic chemical like chlorogenic acid and use it as a 'marker' of identity and quality for 'Echinacea.' What kind of logic or 'science' is that?

With most herbs and foods, we already know which are toxic and which are edible. If we are not sure, we avoid them. There is no need to use any chemical to identify these herbs, unless you want to look for a specific chemical in the food or herb and want to make a drug or dietary chemical out of it. Then, you can disregard everything else and just ingest pectin as your apple and chlorogenic acid when you need 'echinacea' for some health problem. This is getting to sound silly. But this is the conventional wisdom of herbal medicine per the pharmaceutical industry's drug logic. Realistically, we have already been getting some of these chemicals from herbs and foods and using them as dietary (chemical) supplements, bypassing the drug-approval process.

The influence of Western medicine and the pharmaceutical industry on traditional Chinese medicine has been so strong that, during the past century, Chinese herbs and any kind of natural medicine, are reduced to the category of pure chemicals and are treated as such. In fact, there is barely any botanical (or herbal) medicine left which is still treated as it was practiced in the pre-drug era, from antiquity to the early 1800's when morphine was first isolated, and its new synthetic analogs were produced which are much stronger and faster-acting. Unfortunately, they are also becoming more and more toxic. Because of this, Western traditional medicine was steadily moving towards the single-chemical model, exclusively looking for the magic bullet, at first in natural remedies, then in synthetic versions of their natural counterparts, and now in downright synthetics. During these two centuries, Chinese medicine was still largely practiced the traditional way until about 60 years ago, when Western influence rapidly started to intensify. Fast forward to the past ten to twenty years, commercial motives helped to drive Chinese medicine towards active principles (or any chemical with some specific measurable activity). The primary reason was the lack of appropriate scientific technology to deal with them as complex herbs and formulas per se. Another reason was the much easier and more profitable handling of Chinese herbs as some easily analyzed chemicals (whether active or only as marker chemicals). Because of the inability to precisely define Chinese herbs (or any herb) as opposed to pure chemicals, the trend over the past two decades was simply to pick some chemical in the herb, which is easily analyzable and quantifiable, and arbitrarily assign that to represent the herb and call that scientific. Since at least something was now analyzable in the herb, it became readily accepted by scientific experts; now they thought herbs could be 'scientifically defined,' albeit only one chemical out of hundreds or thousands present is analyzed. But, is using pectin as the marker of identity and quality for apple scientific; or chlorogenic acid as marker of identity and quality for 'echinacea' logical? Furthermore, with some herbs, certain chemicals may even be patentable for their specific actions to prevent others (e.g., herbal practitioners) from using the herbs containing them! The result of such handling of herbs has been an increasing spate of commercial herbal ingredients (with high amounts of these standardized chemicals) from China establishing themselves in the natural products market place. These 'high-quality' herbal extracts containing pure chemicals, after being diluted with excipients (inert carriers) and used in herbal supplements or dietary supplements, are becoming common. Examples include ginseng extracts containing 98% ginsenosides, kudzu root extract with 98% puerarin, and extracts of *huzhang* (Japanese knotweed, aka *Polygonum cuspidatum* root) containing 98% resveratrol, a much touted antioxidant present in grapes and wine, though in trace amounts. These extracts are pure chemicals that no longer co-exist or are co-present with other phytochemicals that normally otherwise are present in the herbs and in their genuine extracts. Our Phyto-True fingerprinting can easily distinguish these kinds of products. If these chemicals are to be used as drugs, they should be labeled as such. In fact, they can be part of the natural therapies that are increasingly used as dietary supplements and also as 'herbal' supplements, at least as far as I am aware of. Since these chemicals are not strangers to our environment since antiquity, they don't have all the unknowns of synthetic chemicals. Intensive testing from scratch, as with synthetic modern drugs, are now not necessary.

However, these new chemical supplements are essentially being used out of tradition; and their parent herbs' known and documented efficacy and safely don't apply. The original TCHM with their documented benefits and safety are not utilized while at the same time they are being turned into nontraditional materials without their original long-use history. Then, decades later when we finally realize our mistake and wake up to the fact that we should first modernize our herbs the right way in order to take advantage of our millennia-old documented treasure, it will be too late. The reason is that we will no longer have the traditional herbs as known and documented for all these thousands of years. With these new herbs already based on newly assumed active chemical(s) or irrelevant ones, our human experience with these <u>new</u> herbs will have to be accumulated all over again, over time.

Consequently, modernization of Chinese medicines without retaining their tradition is simply an expedient way to obtain new drugs from herbs, disregarding the invaluable human experience we have already accumulated since antiquity. We are now getting ourselves into the situation of relearning TCHM therapy all over with new, or at best, modified herbs. These new 'modern' drugs (or misguidedly called 'modernized' Chinese medicines) are not TCHM. They are, rather, new drugs based on some chemicals isolated from the herbs or to which they are arbitrarily standardized in the herbs; but they may have none of the total properties traditionally known for the herbs. However, these natural drugs would be nevertheless safer than synthetics because they have been with us in our environment and in our body since human history began, as opposed to synthetic chemicals that are total strangers to us and to our environment. Still, they are <u>not</u> TCHM.

The subject of traditional Chinese medicine (TCM) is complex. It includes various aspects of healing practice such as herbal medicine (aka materia medica), acupuncture, moxibustion, exercises (incl. tai chi or *taiqi, qigong*, & gong fu), *tuina* (massage), *tieda* (trauma medicine such as liniments, plasters & bone-setting) and diet therapy with foods and tonic herbs, among others. It has been practiced since ancient times, with documentations dating back around 3,500 years. In my two books, unless otherwise specified, TCM, TCHM, Chinese medicine(s), Chinese herbs, Chinese drugs, and other related terms, all mean Chinese materia medica (medical materials), whether they are of plant, animal, mineral, or microbial origin. During the past couple of decades, Western ideas infiltrated Chinese medicine. One of them is applying modern science to herbs, even though it is not the right science we have chosen, yet we proudly call it scientific as if the ancient cultures like Chinese had no science. Furthermore, whatever science that is used for modern drug development and therapy is not the proper science for herbs. Consequently, I was optimistic when the founders of the newly formed organization called Modernized Chinese Medicine International Association (MCMIA) contacted me in late 2000, asking me to help them to bring experts from America to their first International Conference that was officially named the First International Conference and Exhibition of the Modernization of Chinese Medicine (ICMCM). I agreed to help them, provided there were no other independent or duplicate efforts from their other international advisors without my being first informed so that I would not waste time with duplicate efforts on our end. They agreed and appointed me as International Advisor to handle the task of inviting American and Canadian experts to be speakers at the conference. I didn't physically send out the invitations; I just talked to friends and colleagues, saying that they should expect official invitations to come from the Conference. Of the fifteen or so experts I talked to and invited to the Conference, about a dozen accepted and were at the Conference. They were all relevant experts, including Dr. Paul Coates, the Director of the Office of Dietary Supplements, who was invited to be the keynote speaker. The other prominent speakers included Dr. Roger Williams (Executive VP & CEO of United States Pharmacopeia), Michael McGuffin (President of American Herbal Products Association), Mark Blumenthal (Founder & Executive Director of American Botanical Council), and Dr.

Richard Ko (California Department of Health Services, now consultant in natural products).

The Conference was held in March 14-17, 2002. I co-chaired a session on "Modernizing Chinese Medicines: Practical Issues" with Dr. Brad Lau, one of the founders of MCMIA. Speakers in our session included Prof. Pei-Shan Xie (Drug Analyst-in-Chief, Guangzhou Institute for Drug Control), Dr. Roger Williams, Greg Pennyroyal (President, Growing Medicine Inc.), Roy Upton (Executive Director, American Herbal Pharmacopoeia) and myself. There were 10 sessions and most of them were on commercialization, marketing, distribution, regulations, quality, and standard-setting issues, among other topics. We all each presented our papers. The trade-show part was very well attended. But the technical part was overwhelmingly oriented towards commerce, including regulations. Nevertheless, with the big-name experts I was bringing in from America, MCMIA was able to match them with some big names from Hong Kong, China, and elsewhere. Hence, it was also able to get funding from the Hong Kong government and many commercial and academic sponsors.

The Conference was a success beyond the founders' wildest expectations. That helped them launch at least one more comparable conference that I know of, and many more exhibitions and scientific seminars of considerably smaller scope. In the banquet that followed and in appreciation of my efforts in their successful Conference, I was presented by the chief founder of MCMIA with a 12-inch by 8-inch glass plaque, perhaps an inch thick, weighing about 7 or 8 pounds. Etched at the bottom were the MCMIA logo both in Chinese and English, my full Chinese name Leung Yuk-Sing, with the Chinese inscription of "Bridge to Traditional Chinese Medicine" underneath. I am sure that was a genuine gesture on the part of the founders, especially since my efforts were all free of charge to them because I only did it for the advancement (modernization) of Chinese medicine, thinking that it was worth a shot to have a chance to promote true modernization of Chinese medicine. I did it again for another year, though, by then, I had lost my confidence and enthusiasm for that group to handle true modernization. Most of them were only interested in making commercial connections and looking for the easiest ways to make money from Chinese herbs in whatever forms. During the past 15 years since my involvement with modernization, many of the stakeholders used the connections from the original two ICMCM's of 2002 and 2003 to strike deals between America and China. Nothing has changed in terms of modernizing Chinese medicine. Instead, more and more herbal extracts coming in from China are pure chemicals sold as 'highly purified' extracts. One of the experts I brought in for the Second ICMCM is a friend, Frank Jaksch, who is a founder of Chromadex. He has recently been in the news promoting some nutritional chemical supplement in Hong Kong, partnering with the Watsons chain. I believe he is one of the few technical experts who understands the concept of true modernization of Chinese herbs. However, being also a good businessman he hasn't figured out a way to make money from genuine herbal products yet. And, typical of my personality, my one-track mind was on true modernization from the beginning. The name MCMIA attracted my attention sixteen or seventeen years ago. I only recently realized the brochure of the first ICMCM 2002, had a subtitle of "Commercialization of Chinese Medicine" under the title "First International Conference and Exhibition of the Modernization of Chinese Medicine." No wonder it was mostly a trade show and the experts I brought to the Conference from America were simply used to boost the legitimacy and prestige of the Conference (and Exhibition) for marketing purposes. I don't actually remember much about the second Conference because, since the first one, I had written this organization off as having any impact on true modernization of Chinese medicine. I did it again just to be sure I didn't miss the slightest chance of getting into real discussions of true modernization. But to my disappointment, my first instinct was correct. Now, after at least 15 years, I still have not seen any progress in bringing true TCHM and formulas to complement our modern health care. All we have is the more and more sophisticated marketing of chemicals from Chinese herbs as dietary supplements and even as 'herbal' supplements.

Furthermore, during the past 20 years, much work has been done on traditional Chinese medicine in Asia, Australia, Europe, and America. Unfortunately, practically all the efforts have been spent based on the pharmaceutical industry's drug model and none has taken our complex human body into consideration as anything but another natural product, namely, a single entity. Nor was the ramification of a single synthetic chemical drug versus a complex herbal medicine ever seriously considered. [see **Chapter 12: What's Wrong...**] Incidentally, in Issue **#21 (July/August, 1999)** of **LCHN**, now republished as **Are Drugs Better Than Herbs?** I had already published a piece titled *Modernization of traditional herbal medicine – What does it mean?* That was reprinted in **Functional Foods & Nutraceuticals**, p. 38, 40, June 2003, retitled *Modernization of Herbal Medicine is Not 'Pharmaceuticalization'*. In that piece, I pointed out most of the key issues involved in the proper modernization of Chinese medicine.

However, I didn't address the potential benefits of why we need to consider, in seriousness, traditional medicines that have millennia of human experience. This involves three different entities: synthetic chemicals versus natural herbal medicines versus the human body. The last (our body), although besides being macroscopically and visually a single entity on the outside, is in fact an extremely complex living system with billions of chemicals, cells, tissues, and other parts inside, existing together in a well-coordinated manner. It is by no means a scientifically single entity. [see **Chapter 12: What's Wrong...**]

For over 40 of my 55 years of scientific training and career, I was always an 'active-principle' person, thinking in terms of active chemicals, fixating on looking for an active principle of a botanical or herb. I didn't start to realize there was a big flaw in our handling of so-called natural products until we had to deal with herbal supplements – a class of plant materials (herbs) that started to be regulated as food in 1994, yet since day one, we have been treating them as drugs. As I have explained this earlier in both of my **LCHN** and my **Memoir**, especially in the above-mentioned chapter, true modernization of traditional medicine is doable only after we realize that the pharmaceutical industry's way will only continue to lead traditional medicine (e.g., TCHM) down the wrong path, namely, to yield more toxic chemical drugs for our health care. All modernization efforts so far are nothing but drug discovery and development efforts, using herbal medicines as a raw material. They are not modernized traditional medicine!

CHAPTER 14

What Should We Do With Our Invaluable Herbal Treasure?

Besides my personal history, I have spent most of my time telling you how I feel about our health care around the world, especially in my birth country, Hong Kong, and my adopted country, the United States. And I have given you my reasons. In this chapter, I want to tell you what I think we should do.

There has been too much politicking and cronyism among scientists in government and nongovernment institutions during the past sixty to eighty years. I have had the chance to observe them during most of my professional career. Our modern drug development and therapy are stuck in a rut, leading to nowhere. Despite many innovations and new discoveries in the drug development field, there have been no real breakthroughs comparable to the Wonder Drug era of antibiotics of the 1930's. All we have to show is the pharmaceutical industry's way of continuing to try to develop new drugs that beget new diseases, and these new diseases in turn require new drugs to treat, in a vicious cycle. I think this vicious cycle was officially started on April 11, 2017 when the first new drug, valbenazine, was officially approved by our FDA for treating a drug-induced disorder called tardive dyskinesia (delayed involuntary body movements). This disease has been caused by the toxic side-effects of years of taking psychotic, gastrointestinal, and anti-epileptic drugs. [see **Chapter 13: Proper Modernization...**] This news came and went like business as usual. But I am certain that other such new drugs will follow to help the drug industry to live its recently realized dream.

All this despite the fact that we have many alternative options available just in the drug-therapy area alone, not to mention the alternatives in nutrition and in true disease-prevention that have only been barely started. The alternative areas I am going to talk about span across three areas. I believe they will eventually replace the vicious cycle of synthetic drugs, and in half the time it has taken pharmaceutical companies to bring us to our current miserable *status quo* of toxic drugs.

The pharmaceutical industry has already had its chance over a period of sixty to eighty years to try to provide us with their new drugs! The end result they have so far gotten us is this: increasingly more new diseases and misery for us consumers, but perpetual self-generated income for itself whether or not its drugs work or whether we want or need them. There are many reasons that have brought us to our current undesirable state of affairs. One of the most responsible is the financial incentive. To me, it seems to spawn all that is wrong with our sciences in health care, more appropriately called sick care. A tiny minority of our population seems to control the money, power, and hence resources to dictate what the rest of the world have to do to keep themselves healthy or alive.

Nevertheless, despite this depressing minority control of our health care, I still have faith in the decency of the rest of my fellow human-beings, otherwise I would have given up years ago and would have just let my thoughts and opinions lie. Unfortunately, a few of my friends and colleagues have done just that, abandoning the herbal field and happily and successfully pursuing other unrelated businesses without fanfare. However, as a discerning and experienced scientist, I think at least I can express my opinions, based on what I have seen and considered wrong over the fifty plus years of my professional career. At least I owe the world (especially my mentor, friends, and family who have helped shape my person) and our grandchildren and theirs, this much. Perhaps there are like-minded people like me, but with power and resources, to carry on the work necessary to preserve our inherited herbal treasure and to simultaneously break the vicious drug cycle to free fellow-consumers to adopt true natural health care.

Contrary to the opinions of most scientific and medical professionals that drug therapy is scientific, it is, in fact, **not**! The drug development part can be highly scientific. But once a drug enters the human body, there is nothing scientific when it tries to find its way to some targeted object (receptor, enzymes, or other countless chemicals) to resolve a diseased condition supposedly caused by this target. Without precise guidance, it has to find its way to the target, wading through millions of chemicals and cells on its way to its destination. This drug therapy process is not as simple as shooting a clear target, with no interference in between. At best, it's like shooting a moving target or a target blocked by many flying objects. And there is no specific guidance from anyone there to take it to the assumed target to neutralize the disease it has caused.

This drug-therapy scenario is no different than that with an herb, even though the latter is a multi-chemical entity, except for two things: (1) as opposed to a pure-chemical drug, the herb itself contains countless chemicals (many still unidentified) which have been with us on earth since antiquity and have evolved together with our body; and (2) unlike a typical modern synthetic drug with absolutely no safe human-use history, all of our herbs, along with their contained chemicals, have some human-use history that we have accumulated from the dawn of human history. So, drug therapy is no different from herbal therapy. Both processes happen inside our body. The difference lies in the experience of either therapeutic entity (a complex herb or a simple chemical) when it enters our body and interacts with the latter's complex living contents. With a synthetic drug that suddenly appears as a new entity on our planet, when it interacts with our body, we have absolutely no idea what it will do to our body. Responsible scientists make sure it is first tested *in vitro, in vivo*, and in animals, to insure it is at least safe enough that it has not killed any animals, before starting to try it on humans. Only then, its first human experience begins. Even after up to 20 years of clinical trial in humans and finally approved for human use, its real full human experience only starts then. Some drugs are withdrawn from the market some years later because we find them too toxic to continue.

When you compare mere decades of human use of synthetic drugs with millennia of human use of herbs or natural chemicals, I think you can appreciate the different degrees of experience of safety and efficacy between these two entities, namely, synthetic drugs versus natural therapeutics (i.e., herbs & natural chemicals). Hence, I propose we do the following, preferably after reviewing the three scenarios in the **Introduction** and **Chapter 12: What's Wrong with Drugs and Herbal Supplements.**

Screening of true herbal supplements among current dietary supplements. Many of the current 'herbal' supplements on the market are anything but herbal. Two such products with the exact same herbal ingredients on their labels from two or more different manufacturers (or brands) are most likely very different. The major reasons have been explained many times throughout my **Memoir** and **LCHN**, as well as elsewhere in my other writings. They have caused consumers and all of us dearly. Yet 'herbal' supplements are still readily available which have no herbal elements in them, as discovered by the New York Attorney General a few years ago. [see **Introduction** & 'serendipity' in **Glossary**] Nor would they provide consumers with any traditional health benefits. I do not see this situation changing for another ten or fifteen years, as I have already been trying to effect change over a period of more than 25 years. My last e-letter to my colleagues in high places in government, industry, and academia was almost five years ago; unfortunately, nothing has happened. [see **Introduction**]. At my age, I can't wait for another five or ten years. That is why I am appealing to you, the consumers. We can easily take some of the suspicious products on the market and fingerprint them to show their differences and provide you with their results on my blog (**http://ayslcorp.com/blog/**) so that you would know what products to avoid. This would save you money and keep purveyors of herbal supplements on their toes. This can be started within months after my books (**Memoir** & **LCHN**) are published, not another 25 years. I am planning to use 75% of the gross profit from the sales of this book to do this.

At the same time, I'll continue to advocate the proper modernization of traditional Chinese medicine and to save it so that new herbal supplements can be produced properly from modernized TCHM, based on well-known formulas documented throughout Chinese history. (see **Chapter 13: Proper Modernization...**) Hopefully, I can interest some bright minds of the younger generations who can see beyond the misapplied pharmaceutical technologies to pick up the baton to assume leadership.

Production of modernized Chinese herbal formulas as genuine herbal supplements. Even though we already have the mechanism provided by the DSHEA to sell herbal supplements using any kind of nontoxic herbs, the resulting products are mostly some form of irrelevant chemical-based supplements or modern chemicals or drugs. They are not genuine herbal supplements that are supposedly being regulated as foods. To achieve true herbal supplements would take a few years to start, after we have first reset our thinking regarding chemical drugs versus herbal supplements or food. We have to treat TCHM as food or close to food, but not as pharmaceuticals (drugs or chemicals). The Phyto-True system can provide the basics to connect true TCHM, as traditionally used and documented, with this new class of herbal supplements I am proposing. The basics of the Phyto-True system were published in 2010 (see **Glossary**). Together with the technical information in these books (**Memoir** & **LCHN**), they can serve as the first step in disrupting the vicious cycle of toxic-drugs-beget-new-diseases which has been established and perpetuated by the pharmaceutical industry and its associates. There are some such traditional Chinese formulas already available from China and Hong Kong. Some of them have been around for over a hundred years. My concern is that, since some of the scientists in charge of the Chinese Pharmacopoeia are mostly trained by Western drug technologies, they may not have the true nature of Chinese herbs in their view. By the time someone with resources and power decides to truly modernize TCHM and entrusts the task to these scientists, they may go right back to the Western-drug way. By doing so, this valuable world treasure for sure would be lost forever and destined to rest in historic museums. Ideally, we should first modernize TCHM and then produce traditional tried-and-true herbal formulas. But it may be too slow to convert some of the 'modernized' herbs like cured fo-ti (*zhiheshouwu*) back to its traditional form. Fortunately, some of the well-known Chinese formulas are already available as herbal supplements. They can continue to be sold (but with their unique fingerprints) while at the same time we can act to prevent more TCHM from being converted to misguided 'modernized' forms. Although the latter may be standardized to an easily analyzable chemical (thus 'modernized' and 'scientific'), this chemical may often have no relevance to its parent TCHM. For example, ginsenosides don't represent ginseng (Asian, American, or others) and are only one of many major types of important chemicals in it. The others include polysaccharides (carbohydrates), sterols (steroids), peptides, polypeptides, vitamins, pectin, and triterpenes, among many others. The use of ginsenosides as marker compounds for 'ginseng' is strictly a way to market ginseng as if it were a drug easily measurable by chemical analyses, hence considered 'scientific' by consumers and many scientists. However, herbal supplements are not drugs, as I have repeatedly stressed. Since the DSHEA was passed in 1994, they are regulated as foods, but have, since day one, been treated as drugs (i.e., chemicals).

For Western herbs, this has not been a problem because we analyze them for their chemicals and use these chemicals as drugs. Unlike Chinese herbal medicine, Western herb use does not have an extensive, continuous documentation. Around the time when the modern drug era started 150 years or so ago, the field was known as materia medica (medical materials) that is a forerunner of pharmacognosy. The science of materia medica and pharmacognosy has always been focused on turning natural materials (e.g., herbs) into 'modern' drugs, meaning chemical drugs. That is Western medicine, usually called "modern" medicine. I am no historian or expert in the evolution or history of Western medicine. But it seems that, from around the time natural chemicals (e.g. morphine) started to be used alone (isolated from plants) as new drugs, the raw herbs (e.g., opium poppy) have been left behind. And materia medica was somehow transitioned into modern chemical drugs. At first, these modern drugs were new natural chemicals such as morphine, salicin, and ephedrine. Then, synthetic modifications of these natural chemicals started to appear, including aspirin. As far as I know, once we find a chemical in a Western herb with some similar property as its source herb, we simply try to turn that into a new chemical drug. Then, the herb is largely abandoned. Most of the Western population has since gravitated towards modern drugs, leaving a tiny minority of true traditional herbalists to carry on the Western herbal tradition. Consequently, unlike with Chinese herbs, there has not been any traditional way for scientists to look at Western herbs other than through the pharmaceutical industry's chemical lens. Even up to this day, most scientists such as pharmacognosists and natural product chemists view natural materials as natural chemicals or drugs. They never had to distinguish the 'natural products' they studied because in their mind these eventually would all end up being some chemicals or drugs anyway. [see **Preface** & **LCHN-32** for more detailed explanation of pharmacognosy] Consequently, when herbal supplements first appeared 25 years ago, they didn't know how to deal with them, except to treat them as chemicals, hence drugs. Applying the technologies developed specifically for chemical drugs on herbs (especially Chinese herbs) had produced most of our problems whenever we try to deal with herbs. These are still unresolved. In this book, I am trying to introduce my disruptive concept of a true alternative therapeutic system that can accompany, complement and replace part of our current synthetic-drug system.

Since one of the most developed traditional herbal systems is Chinese medicine, it can be used as a model for <u>new source of herbal supplements, natural therapeutics, and natural drugs</u>. For decades, I have been outspoken on the proper way to utilize our natural therapeutic resources and to assure TCHM be appropriately preserved and modernized. I was among two other experts, Dr. Richard Ko and Greg Pennyroyal, invited to brief USP's top executives and technical experts (about six or seven of them altogether) at its US headquarters shortly before USP's decision to open an office and a laboratory in China around 2005. It finally did so. I haven't kept track of its activities in China. But as far as I know there hasn't been any earth-breaking news on USP activities from China in recent years. And there has been no sign of Chinese herbs being handled any differently than by the usual pharmaceutical way – analyzing their chemicals as if herbs are simply arbitrarily chosen chemicals. Therefore, I am still trying to persuade my colleagues to reset their thinking and to start treating Chinese herbs the right way that will finally give us appropriate results. Simultaneously, I am also appealing to the general public because of its unbiased mind.

While pursuing true modernization and at the same time trying to prevent the continued misguided modification of TCHM with irrelevant drug technologies, we can still produce and market true herbal supplements. These include the tried-and-true Chinese herbal formulas that have been used safely and documented for centuries and millennia, as well as genuine extracts of Western herbs with fingerprints other than some chemical markers. The key is a total fingerprint with or without specific chemical markers.

Production of modern drugs from natural chemicals. Our current *status quo* of modern drug therapy is too entrenched for us to do anything about. Not much can be done in the short term because the system is so set up that like the human body, disturbance in one part reverberates throughout the rest, causing chaos. Nobody indebted to the pharmaceutical industry is going to do anything differently and voluntarily since they all have been doing the same thing for many decades. I don't know how many percent of our citizens are beneficiaries of the pharmaceutical industry, but we all pay exorbitant prices for drugs it demands, to support its drug therapy that can be a vicious cycle for us consumers. The action will have to come from consumers, taxpayers, and the rest of the citizenry who are not indebted to drug companies.

One thing we can do is to make new safer modern drugs by first starting to produce them from non-synthetic, natural sources such as chemicals from TCHM. There are countless of these chemicals recorded in the traditional Chinese herbal literature, as most of the research on Chinese herbs during the past hundred years has been on their contained chemicals. For example, just take ginseng alone, American or Asian. There are dozens of ginsenosides present in it, not including additional dozens of closely related compounds present in the leaf of a gourd plant (*Gynostemma pentaphyllum*). Many of them have varied biological properties when tested alone, such as ginsenoside Rb-1 (tranquilizing) versus ginsenoside Rg-1 (stimulating). Any one of them can be explored for its specific bioactivity that can be turned into a milder and possibly more effective modern drug. Although these are all chemicals, they still have been part of our existence and ecosystem, not like synthetics. They will not need all the extensive testing as being applied to totally new and unpredictable synthetic chemicals. And their cost would also be much lower than most current OTC drugs. [see **Chapter 12: What's Wrong...**]

The isolated natural chemicals now readily available (e.g., from China & India) can be developed and marketed as dietary (or chemical) supplements so that they are not confused with true herbal supplements or with synthetic chemical drugs. Many of them are already being marketed in America. However, they are still chemical drugs, except they have been with us since ancient times and their toxicities are bound to be fewer. At the end, they will return to our environment from which they had come. Hence, they are environmentally much friendlier than any synthetics.

The natural chemicals described above are more complicated and involved than herbs and herbal formulas (the true herbal supplements), but they still can be turned into safer and more reliable natural modern drugs that can become a new industry to compete with conventional synthetic pharmaceuticals. There are many clues in TCHM which can lead to other modern natural drugs. These cannot be obtained from the mostly unknown and uncertain synthetics whose history of contact and interaction with humans is no more than 100 years, as opposed to millennia for herbal therapeutics. Examples of natural drugs include the antimalarial artemisinin from sweet annie (*Artemisia annua*) and many other natural chemicals such as huperzine A, oleanolic acid, sitosterol, resveratrol, and berberine, to name just a few. All have specific biological effects that we seek. A whole new business of natural drugs with less unpredictable toxic-effects and centuries or millennia of human experience, plus their lower cost, can only improve the physical, mental, and financial status of the entire health and wellness system.

CHAPTER 15

Glossary and Abbreviations

Active principle – an active chemical in an herb or plant found to be the chemical responsible for most of the traditional herb's sought-after properties. There are many other active chemicals in plants/herbs but they may have nothing to do with a major part of the herbs' traditionally known activities.

AHP – American Herbal Pharmacopoeia, an organization modelled after the USP/NF, except it is strictly for botanicals.

Amah – a live-in nanny and maid in Asia.

Analog – a sister compound or chemical with similar chemical structure as another, being different only in a certain aspect of it.

Angiosperms – flowering plants like apples, oranges and lilies, etc.

Anthraglycoside – short form for anthraquinone glycoside. A glycoside is made up of 2 units, a sugar (glucose, mannose, etc.) and a non-sugar compound; in this case, the non-sugar part is derived from anthracene (from coal tar used for making dyes) which in its oxidized form is a quinone, called anthraquinone. These anthraglycosides are widely present in nature, e.g., cascara, senna, and drug aloe (though only in traces in the gel). They are called stimulant laxatives.

Big Pharma – Pharmaceutical companies as a whole.

Big Pharma & Company (BPCo) – Big Pharma and its interdependent associates that include the medical profession, other associated healthcare professionals, the insurance industry, indebted politicians, lobbyists, and others that benefit from the business activities of the pharmaceutical industry.

CHM – Chinese herbal medicine.

CM – Chinese medicine.

CMM – Chinese materia medica, Chinese medical materials, Chinese drug, CM, CHM, TCHM.

CNS – central nervous system

CP – Chinese Pharmacopoeia or Pharmacopoeia of the People's Republic of China; a government organization for setting standards of chemical drugs and Chinese herbs.

Decoction – in general, boiling with water; more specifically, extraction made by boiling herbs with roughly 2 to 3 times the amount of water until down to ½ - 1/3 the amount, usually repeated once. Normally, the herbs are first soaked in water for a short time (e.g., 30 min) before heating.

DSHEA – Dietary Supplement Health and Education Act passed in October 1994.

DSLD – Dietary Supplement Label Database – see Chapter 11.

Excipient – inert material that serves as filler, carrier, etc. in finished products; it can be a marc, rice hulls, cellulose powder, propylene glycol, and many others.

Extract strengths – the strengths of traditional whole extracts are expressed by ratios such as 2X or 2:1, meaning starting with 4 kg of dried herb extracted exhaustively with a suitable solvent, such as water or alcohol (ethanol, methanol, mixtures, or others) to yield 2 kg of extract. For any particular solvent, the more it extracts from the herb, the lower the strength of the final extract; and vice versa. This is traditionally done. A high-strength extract is not necessarily better than a lower-strength extract. For example, lycium (goji) berries have lots of water- soluble extractives (extractable materials) including sugars, polysaccharides, amino acids, and others. If you use hot water to extract them exhaustively, you may get up to 50% of extractives removed, resulting in an extract that is a 2X concentrate or of 2:1 strength. If one wants to cheat and claim higher strength and higher price for his lycium berry extract under the assumption that higher (or bigger) is better, he can achieve this in 2 ways. He can extract the berries not exhaustively but rather quickly, getting 25% of extractives instead of 50% out. Now, out of 4 kg of dried berries he only gets 1 kg, resulting in a 4X (4:1) extract. Since the marc remaining still has a lot of polysaccharides, betaine, taurine, and flavonoids, and can be further extracted with water to get another sizable amount of extractives. This can be standardized to any of these chemicals and be sold as a 'standardized' extract. I think it may even be legal with standardized extracts, as few companies would care how they are obtained as long as it meets some standardized chemical content. But this is one of the practices that would eventually obliterate Chinese medicine.

Extracts – the terminology used in the botanical (herbal) extracts industry has changed little over the past 100 years, except the numbers used in expressing their strengths. A strength of 1:3 (originally used to mean 3X concentrate) has been gradually changed to 3:1 that is now more commonly used. Be sure to ask the manufacturer which strength it means because the confusion is common. There are various types of extracts: native, solid, powdered, fluid, tincture, infusion, etc. Native extracts are right out of the kettle (or extractor) before anything is done to it. It is usually a thick viscous liquid, sometimes also called solid extract even though it is not a solid. When excipients are added to it to standardize it to a certain strength, it becomes a standardized solid extract (2:1 or 3:1, etc.). Further treatment, such as drying, would yield a powdered extract. Fluidextract is an extract obtained by using a mixture of alcohol and water; its strength usually is 1:1. Tinctures are much weaker than fluidextracts, such as 10% or 0.1:1 strength. Infusions are mostly hot water extracts, e.g., tea, with no further concentration.

Ginsenosides – one of the major types of compounds found in ginseng (e.g., American & Asian) – they are saponin glycosides.

Glycosides – Compounds formed by sugars (e.g., glucose) and sterols or other non-sugar compounds, widely distributed in plants.

Goji – colloquial name used for lycium fruit in marketing; the official Chinese transliteration of lycium fruit is *gouqizi*; the plant itself is *gouqi*.

Gymnosperms – non-flowering plants, like pine trees, spruce trees, and ephedra (*mahuang*) herb, etc.

Healing foods – In the practice of medicine, traditionally both in the East and West, some foods are consider medicine, and vice versa. In TCM, herbs and foods that are used for both purposes are often refer to as tonics or healing foods, such as ginsengs, watercress and astragalus.

HPLC – High-Performance Liquid Chromatography is an analytical technique for analyzing and separating chemical mixtures. A solution of the mixture is introduced onto the top of a column packed with a powder (called adsorbent, appropriate for the chemicals to be separated), followed by a solvent (e.g., alcohol, hexane) that continuously carries the chemicals in the mixture down the tube. These chemicals have different affinities for the adsorbent and hold on to it with different degrees of tightness. Eventually, this solvent will carry them all down the column and they will emerge at the bottom in the solvent one at a time, thus can be recovered separately. Simultaneously, a graph shows a picture of the chemicals emerging at different times from the column, forming a fingerprint (chromatogram) of peaks and valleys.

HPTLC – High-Performance Thin-Layer Chromatography is an analytical technique for analyzing compounds of many kinds on a flat surface coated with a thin layer of a solid, called adsorbent (e.g., silica gel or aluminum oxide) on which a solution of a mixture of chemicals is spotted (as a band) at one end of the plate and dipped into a solvent. The latter rises up the plate by capillary action, carrying the chemicals with different abilities to hold onto the adsorbent up the plate, thus moving at different speeds upward, to form different bands like those in a rainbow. A mixture of components from an herb extract can be separated into distinct bands forming a unique fingerprint. HPTLC's versatility lies in allowing the same mixture of chemicals to be tested in different conditions at the same time, by dipping more than one identical plate with the same spotted bands of the same mixture in different solvents (i.e., conditions), thus affording more precise and accurate results much more economically.

i.g., i.m., i.v., b.i.d., t.i.d. – intra gastric, intramuscular, intravenous, twice-a-day, 3X-a-day, respectively

ICMCM – "International Conference & Exhibition of the Modernization of Chinese Medicine." Note the Exhibition part is not represented in the title, despite the first two conferences I helped organize in Hong Kong were mostly about commercial products as I had believed otherwise.

LCHN – Leung's Chinese Herb News, republished with my Memoir in a single volume renamed, *Are Drugs Better Than Herbs? An Insider's Scientific Look at Drugs and Herbal Supplements*.

Marc – herbal materials after they have been exhaustively extracted with solvents; since it should no longer contain anything active, it is used sometimes as carrier or filler in finished products.

Marker chemical – also called marker compound, is any chemical chosen in an herb to represent the herb (or botanical) because it can be easily analyzed so that it can be arbitrarily assigned to be the herb's marker of identity and quality. However, it may have nothing to do with the herb's properties and actions as traditionally known and documented.

MCMIA – Modernized Chinese Medicine International Association.

Menstruum – extracting solvent that can be water, alcohol, a mixture, etc. Now, not as commonly used.

NCCAM – National Center for Complementary and Alternative Medicine, now renamed National Center for Complementary and Integrative Health (NCCIH), a part of the National Institutes of Health (NIH).

NCCIH – See NCCAM.

NLM – National Library of Medicine.

Nutraceuticals – nutritional chemicals.

ODS – Office of Dietary Supplements.

OTC drugs – Over-The-Counter drugs.

Pharmacognosy – a term used to describe the study of drugs from natural sources; together with pharmacology, they used to be known as materia medica (medical materials); now, it is the study of chemicals or herbs derived from nature, with no clear distinction among them. See **Preface** of this book for more details.

Phytochemicals – chemicals from plants as distinguished from chemical synthesis.

Phytonutrients – broad class of nutrients from plants, including vitamins, established nutrients like some carotenoids and flavonoids, and also many newly discovered chemicals with antioxidant or other properties assumed to have health effects but may not yet proven safe in humans.

Phytopharmaceuticals – drugs from plants.

Phyto-True system – A scientific system that properly deals with complex herbs and complex natural materials or products/herbs which simultaneously takes care of both the modern scientific and the traditional aspects of herbs, including herbal supplements as opposed to identified and well-defined pure chemicals: A.Y. Leung, Tradition- and science-based quality control of traditional Chinese medicine – introducing the Phyto-True system, *J. AOAC International* **93** (5): 1355-1366 (2010)

Polysaccharides – broadly known as carbohydrates consisting of monosaccharides (including single sugars units such as glucose, fructose, mannose, etc.), disaccharides (sucrose, maltose, etc.), and polysaccharides that contain 3 or more units of monosaccharides. Polysaccharides can be very long-chained and are present in most herbs (ginsengs, astragalus, aloe gel, etc.); many of them have regulatory effects on our immune system.

Question 1: How can consumers tell superior from inferior herbal products? They can't, unless there is a universally agreed-upon standard on every herbal material as is currently practiced with pure chemical drugs. But we still can fingerprint the ingredients in them with Phyto-True techniques using multiple tests (HPTLC, HPLC, etc.) so that the fingerprint would show the whole picture where you can see the missing parts if they are not there or extra chemicals that don't belong there. At present (2018), such fingerprinting is not required. Hence, we don't have product consistency in herbal supplements as opposed to chemical drugs. Consequently, we need a competent lab supported by the general public to analyze questionable products to help consumers to decide whether a product is simply a chemical (mixed with carriers or fillers) or a real herbal supplement containing genuine herbal extracts, as claimed.

Question 2: Is there a good source of herbal ingredients? Currently no, because they are mostly standardized against some presumed active chemicals even if they are only a few among other countless chemicals in the herbs, like ginsenosides for ginseng extracts and curcumin for turmeric. Even though they may be all legal, they are mostly arbitrarily selected chemicals, not herbs; and should be sold only as dietary chemicals (dietary supplements) and not as herbal supplements.

Rhizomes – underground stems of plants, sometimes also called runners; they produce roots below and shoots above. They are not roots; for example, the spice or drug, turmeric, is not the root of the Curcuma plant, but its rhizome. The actual root of the turmeric (Curcuma) plant has very different properties and, compared to the spice (i.e., turmeric), it has much less curcumin.

Saponins – Glycosides whose water solutions foam when shaken.

Selective extract – picking out specific chemicals and selectively extract them; it is not a whole extract.

Serendipity – The DNA testing used by the chemist(s) for the New York Attorney General in analyzing finished herbal supplements (incl. ginseng, ginkgo biloba, and Echinacea, among others) is only appropriate for analyzing those containing unprocessed ground herbs. It is not suitable for processed herbal extracts or products, especially those based on some standardized chemicals; in those 'herbal' supplements containing standardized chemicals, the DNA may come only from the carriers or fillers (ground inert herbs or other raw plant materials) because products that only containing these chemicals don't have DNA. Nevertheless, the DNA testing exposed by chance that many 'herbal' products are not true herbal supplements but are based on some standardized chemicals (markers) of herbal extracts, with the rest being inert fillers like rice husks and dried inert herbs.

Standardization – a way to define the identity and quality of herbs (botanicals) by selecting a chemical (or a group of chemicals), often arbitrarily, to represent the particular herb concerned. Since this chemical is known and easily analyzable, it can be set at a certain percentage to be in the herb or its extract so that a product containing it can be consistently made with this chemical within the preset amounts, batch after batch. The question is: what if that chemical does not represent the properties of the herb or extract that also contains many other chemicals, known or unknown? This enables easy commercial adulteration or spiking with the added pure chemical in the particular extract which meets the amount of the standardized chemical but without other herbal chemicals from the herb also present. Examples of such adulteration is common, including adding highly purified 'extracts' such as 98% pure ginseng extract (meaning ginsenosides), 98% pure turmeric extract containing only pure curcumin but without other components also present in turmeric, or 98% resveratrol extract from *Polygonum cuspidatum* or Japanese knotweed. These chemicals have no place as herbal supplements other than being added (spiked) to so-called herbal supplements as label claim; and many of these 'herbal' supplements contain no other herbal elements in them, except the arbitrarily assigned chemical. Currently, these kinds of pure chemicals come mostly from China and India.

Standardized extracts – These are extracts with a certain preset amount of some assumed active chemical that is analyzable so that this amount is always present; but what if that chemical has nothing to do with the traditional properties of the herb? Besides, it is not an herb but a drug, unless this extract is a whole extract of an herb standardized against a chemical present in it in its naturally present state.

TCHM – traditional Chinese herbal medicine, Chinese herbal medicine, traditional Chinese herbs

TCM – Traditional Chinese medicine, a general term that includes CHM, CM, TCHM, CMM, and other practices such as acupuncture, exercise, massage or *tuina*, moxibustion, etc. TCM is also a broad term that includes not just herbs but medicines (drugs) in general, such as therapeutics derived from minerals and animals as well

Testing *in vitro* (in test tube) and *in vivo* (in living matter)

Thermogenic – heat producing; as with some chemicals or drugs that are known to stimulate metabolism to produce heat to 'burn' fats, thus lose weight.

THM – traditional medicine, traditional herbal medicine, traditional herbs

USP/NF (United States Pharmacopeia/National Formulary) – Nonprofit & nongovernment organization that sets standards for drugs, dietary chemicals (vitamins, etc.), and herbs used in pharmaceuticals and dietary supplements.

Whole extract (wholesome) – extracts from which nothing is removed.

Made in the USA
San Bernardino, CA
12 August 2018